A Novel Diet

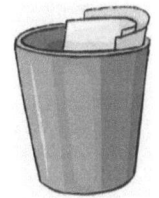

A Novel Diet

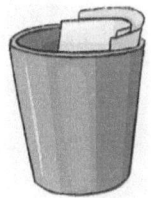

Learn Why You Failed Before
&
How Not To Fail Again

Nikki Lang, M.D.

iUniverse, Inc.
New York Bloomington Shanghai

A Novel Diet
Learn Why You Failed Before & How Not To Fail Again

iUniverse
1663 Liberty Drive
Bloomington, IN 47403
www.iuniverse.com
1-800-Authors (1-800-288-4677)

Because of the dynamic nature of the Internet, any Web addresses or links contained in this book may have changed since publication and may no longer be valid.

You should not undertake any diet/exercise regimen recommended in this book before consulting your personal physician. Neither the author nor the publisher shall be responsible or liable for any loss or damage allegedly arising as a consequence of your use or application of any information or suggestions contained in this book.

ISBN: 978-0-595-44451-9 (pbk)
ISBN: 978-0-595-68951-4 (cloth)
ISBN: 978-0-595-88778-1 (ebk)

Printed in the United States of America

CONTENTS

* **Information contained within dialogue of novel.**

APPENDIX

---

*   **Information contained within dialogue of novel.**

EDITOR'S FOREWORD

When I took on the project of editing *A Novel Diet* in September of 2006, I found the topic interesting, but I never dreamed it would affect my life personally. I was familiar with other diet books, so I didn't expect this one to be any different. I was wrong.

As a book editor and publishing consultant working from home, my daily lifestyle had become akin to that of a sedentary slug in a Texas August. Up to that point, my thirty-foot commute from the bedroom to the office was the best exercise I'd get all day. After my pregnancy with my daughter four years earlier, I had become significantly overweight. Even though I'd lost some weight at one point, I'd eventually gained it all back.

It hadn't been for lack of trying. After my daughter was born, I'd adopted a healthier lifestyle, but I also developed a problem in my right knee that made walking for extended distances painful. So I started practicing yoga to strengthen and stretch my muscles, and get some form of exercise.

I guess it's important to note that I'm a Type A personality that tries to take on multiple tasks at once. I'm perpetually in danger of having so many irons in the fire that none of them light. By the time my daughter was two, I was weighted down with multiple obligations, as usual, and also had a fallout with a primary family member. As you will discover while reading Cheryl's story, emotional implications can hinder accomplishment. For me, this familial fallout had put my already driven, yet exasperating day into full tilt.

In my depressed state, I got by doing only the bare minimum. After a year or so, I wasn't doing yoga at all, nor exercising. I had seen a chiropractor about my knee, though. After receiving treatment for over six months, I had worked up to walking two miles a day. Even though I had enjoyed long-distance running in my teens and early twenties, the walking eventually became just one more mundane task to do in my already overloaded twenty-first century day—and it was boring and monotonous.

As you'll read in *A Novel Diet*, prioritizing time is paramount for weight loss. True to my personality, I had added two college classes to my schedule when I'd first started editing Dr. Lang's book that September. These classes had at least gotten me out of the house and walking more (to and from classes), which I think helped a bit. However, by the time I'd finished my first edit of her book in November, I'd been eating breakfast on a regular basis (Step 2, as you'll discover), working toward eating the five small meals a day (Step 3, Step 4), and taking ballroom dancing lessons with my husband (an activity directed at Step 5). I had taken lessons several years before and loved it. By December, I had lost thirty pounds "without really trying," as I told Dr. Lang.

None of these life changes felt like burdensome additions to my to-do list. Thanks to the changes in my eating habits, I felt a difference in my overall energy level throughout the day. And I loved dancing with my husband; he happily chased me all around the dance floor. As you will discover in this book, it's very beneficial to find an exercise activity you enjoy, and I think that's true. I had plenty of discipline in other areas, but when it came to exercise, Dr. Lang was right: if you really enjoy something, you'll be much more apt to go do it. I needed to play—and dancing was literally just what the doctor ordered.

But then I came down with a bad case of life overload once again, and some of my newfound good habits disappeared. By February of 2007, I'd told Dr. Lang about the weight loss and the subsequent backsliding. Though I'd now edited her book twice, even I had forgotten to apply one of Dr. Lang's biggest principles to my progress: it takes time to create habits. She reminded me that I probably was still implementing many habits I wasn't giving myself credit for doing. Because I hadn't attained the perfect progress my personality wanted to see, I thought I wasn't adhering to the program. However, I was still doing exactly what Dr. Lang's approach emphasizes: developing healthy habits. Sure enough, when I'd thought about it, I was still eating breakfast on a regular basis, and sometimes the smaller meals. I had retained some of those habits, and more importantly, had not gained any weight back!

I have since revised my schedule and dismissed the things that are less important in the long run in exchange for activities that are good for my health and overall lifestyle. I look forward, pleasantly, to more long-term progress. May you enjoy the life-changing process and the genuine results as much as I have.

Thank you, Dr. Lang.

Lori Lisi
May 31, 2007
Author consultant at www.book-proposal.com

TESTIMONIALS

"Dr. Lang's book explains the concepts of changing habits in a way that we can all relate to—baby steps! She speaks on how the average woman, with a busy schedule and a hectic family life, can lose weight. I enjoyed learning the scientific concepts of weight loss in a simple way."
—Paula Dockery
Patient
Warehouse manager
Greenwhich Services, Philadelphia

"I really and truly love this book because I have been struggling with my weight all my adult life, and it hit home! I love how you incorporated the diet modifications, exercise information, and explanation of body chemistry regarding diet—without having it sound so clinical. It was easy to read and understand … and apply to my own lifestyle. I loved the ending … Is there going to be a sequel?"
—Fran Troilo
Account manager
Labcorp, Philadelphia

"I found your book not only entertaining, but informative. I was able to see myself in the character of Cheryl … Everybody likes a story where there is a winner, and we can all see ourselves as such in your book. There are practical solutions … and I'm learning to bring about the changes that I both want and need!"
—Margaretta L. Nicholson
Patient
Licensed practical nurse
Hospital of the University of Pennsylvania

"You know I am a believer. Your book has brought a great change in my life."
—Maria Travaglio
Patient
Bookkeeper
Archdiocese of Philadelphia

"Dr. Lang's book inspired me to lose weight the right way. It seems that five or six small meals a day can make weight loss so much easier because you're not constantly hungry. Understanding all the principles of healthy eating, not just one or two, makes you realize that you don't have to starve yourself, and you don't have to give up your favorite foods. Knowledge is truly the power that can promote a healthy lifestyle and eating in a way that is comfortable for you. I would recommend this book to anyone who's looking to return to his or her ideal weight. It worked for me. I lost 25 pounds, and it wasn't difficult."
—Cynthia Lawson
Pharmaceutical representative
Astra Zenaca

STOP! READ ME FIRST

If you've read other diet books before, then you know that all the well-known diets take one or two basic principles of weight loss, like eating no carbs or eating every three hours, and turn it into a book. These principles have been around for years and years; they are not original concepts. But because most people embark on a diet with so little knowledge, they believe they've just come across a brilliant new method that might finally work for them.

Even the Atkins Diet was not original. Dr. Robert Atkins popularized a classic concept first noted by William Banting in *Letter on Corpulence*, originally published in 1869. The basic tenets of the diet—eating only protein and fat—were scoffed at by the modern medical community and certainly not readily accepted until recent years.

All these diets, whether it's the newest Three-Hour Diet, Volumetrics, South Beach, or the Glycemic Index Diet, are based on well-known, well-worn nutritional precepts expanded into a book.

I have covered these principles in the following pages. Each is given about one chapter or less, and each diet overlaps the others in some ways. For example, the Glycemic Index Diet is loosely based on Atkins's principles of not raising blood sugar too much. South Beach is also based on Atkins and/or the Glycemic Index Diet principles, adding to it a decrease in high-fat foods containing saturated and trans fats. This diet keeps the heart healthier while also decreasing calorie counts.

Please don't think I am putting these diets down; they all work, if you stick to their principles faithfully. The problem is adhering to any one of them exclusively without the knowledge of the others.

Read these diets, understand them, and move on. We all want a quick fix (as Cheryl, the main character in my novel, learns). We read one book once and think we have sufficient knowledge to do the job. How well would we perform in our careers if we read just one book? Most of our jobs take a lifetime of study and experience to do well.

Eating to be trim and healthy is a difficult job. The more knowledge you have, the easier it will become.

"But plenty of people stay slim without any knowledge at all," you might say. "Why is it so much easier for some people to stay thin than others? Knowledge must not be the only factor."

Well, there is no doubt that genes play a role. Some medical conditions can influence metabolism and appetite. People who suffer from a genetic disorder called Prader-Willi Syndrome would eat themselves to death if permitted. They are deficient in a type of hormone that allows for the sensation of satiety. They never feel full—they keep eating. I would venture to say that we all have varying amounts of these appetite-regulating hormones.

Environmental, social, and emotional factors also help to govern the differences in our approach to eating.

One of the many principles I've learned, as a physician, is that the human population truly follows a bell-shaped curve. For those who are unfamiliar with this curve, it is a graph that takes the shape of a bell when we plot almost any statistic. No matter what behavior or illness is graphed, we all fall somewhere on that statistical curve. Moving our position on that curve can be difficult. Change is difficult.

If you grow up in a household that generally eats healthy as a matter of course, you may develop good habits early on. If you have a traumatic or stressful childhood, you may learn to eat for comfort or not eat due to anxiety. We're all different and clearly not created equal. As Bill Gates recently said in a speech to college students, "Life isn't fair. Get over it!"

So, yes, some of the cards you've been dealt may not be the best, but knowledge, small changes, and patience can influence much of that. If anyone tells you it's easy to lose weight and keep it off using their method or pill or whatever, they're lying. It's not easy, because change is not easy. We human beings are resistant to change. Losing weight and keeping it off requires permanent changes. Pills and diets don't provide that. A combination of small, easy changes can ultimately make huge differences.

You must, however, know which changes to make. If you've been on numerous diets in the past, you have some of the necessary information, but you may also have some misinformation. You need to integrate that information and learn how to use it.

This book can do that for you. The text sections at the end of each appropriate novel chapter will help you understand and reinforce what you need to do. As you implement very small easy changes, you'll begin to realize that there really is a sort of magic embedded in this book. But that magic is really about you—your attitude, beliefs, knowledge, and understanding.

Chapter One

February 2005

Cheryl stared into the undersized dressing-room mirror. Tears welled up in her eyes, blurring her vision and slowly sliding down her cheeks. All five gowns she'd tried on might as well have been burlap sacks, not designer dresses.

Cheryl yanked off the last dress and stared angrily at the sweaty rolls of fat glistening in her reflection. She grabbed her sides as though she were wearing a spare tire, desperately trying to shed it. When the stubborn mass wouldn't budge, she started to sob aloud and collapsed onto the worn dressing-room bench with her face in her hands. In utter frustration, she kicked one of the garments from underfoot, causing it to land in a heap in the corner.

From a few stalls over, Cheryl heard her friend, Teresa, call out. "Hey, Cheryl. Hurry up, we've got to get going. We're supposed to meet the gang in five minutes at Friday's. We're going to be really late. Cheryl? Hey, Cheryl!"

Cheryl silently tried to catch her breath and regain enough composure to respond. Suddenly, Teresa was banging on the dressing-room door. "Come on, we're gonna be late!"

"You go ahead," Cheryl managed to choke out, hiding her distress. "I'll catch up with you."

"Are you sure? I can wait."

"No, no, you go ahead. I'll be there in a bit."

"Well, if you're sure it's okay." Seconds later, Teresa was gone.

Cheryl sat for a while, drying her tears and trying to figure out what had gotten into her. She had never felt such despair before. Hell, she'd been fat for almost fifteen years—why was today any different? So what if she was going to someone else's wedding and not her own? That was nothing unusual. Thirty-two years old and still single, she'd watched most of her high school friends get married without such an emotional reaction.

But now, she finally felt like giving up on her appearance. Why bother buying a new expensive dress? Anything that didn't highlight her big belly just looked like a tent on her. Why not just wear something old? Nobody'd know the difference. No one looked at her anyway. She thought about not going to the wedding, but

Wendy had been a good friend for many years. It would be more work explaining her absence than going. Maybe she'd just treat herself to a new pair of shoes and handbag, and wear the dress from Carol's wedding party.

That problem solved, she dried her tears, got dressed, and headed off to Friday's.

*   *   *

Cheryl hadn't always been fat. Up until age seventeen, she had been almost too thin. She'd always been active and loved to dance. With her bubbly personality, she had been the life and soul of the party. She had really known how to dress, too, and had enjoyed showing off the latest fashions. With her then lithe body and athleticism, she had been a shoo-in at cheerleading tryouts.

It was safe to say that Cheryl was probably one of the most popular girls at school—before tragedy wiped away that cheerful girl everyone had known. Cheryl's little sister, Joy, was hit by a car and killed, and the person Cheryl had been disappeared with her.

Cheryl had been babysitting her sister one day after school while her mother was gone grocery shopping. She sat outside on the front stoop, watching Joy play with a basketball. Joy, who had decided she was going to be the first famous female basketball player, was practicing her dribbling, bouncing the ball every which way. She frequently shouted, "Cheryl, watch this!" or "I bet you can't do this!"

The phone rang, and Cheryl jumped up and ran inside the house to answer it, thinking it might be Teresa calling her back. No, it wasn't her closest friend. It was an annoying telemarketer, and it only took Cheryl a moment to realize it and hang up. As she walked back outside, she heard an alarming screech of tires and a sickening thud. Frantically, she glanced around for Joy, who was no longer on the sidewalk. Cheryl looked up just in time to see a nondescript car take off like a bat out of hell.

She heard a shrill cry of pain, not realizing it was her own as she viewed the crushed body of her adored little sister lying in the middle of the street. She ran into the street, still wailing, still hoping. Blood oozed from Joy's ear, and her little body lay at an odd angle to her head and neck. Her basketball was a few feet away, under a car across the street from their house. Cheryl felt the sudden urge to vomit and instinctively turned away so she wouldn't throw up on her sister. She collapsed to her knees, puking and sobbing next to Joy. One of the neighbors saw what was happening and called the police.

The officers arrived at the same time that Cheryl's mother, Charlotte, appeared back from the grocery store. Cheryl was so hysterical that she wasn't making any sense at all. Charlotte took one look at what was in front of her and become equally distraught. The police tried in vain to calm them down. An ambulance came, but everyone knew it was too late for Joy.

Although Cheryl had gotten only the briefest glimpse of the escaping car, she had enough wherewithal to note the license-plate number, which she related to the police between sobs. The police put out an APB with a description of the car, which was found the next day, abandoned not more than twenty-five minutes from the house. Although investigators were able to get several good DNA samples from the stolen car from cigarettes in the ashtray, they never did find a match in any of the databases. It was still an open case.

In the months after, Cheryl tried to avoid thinking about Joy. But reminders of her little sister were everywhere. Cheryl began avoiding friends. Their good-intentioned inquiries about how she was doing would simply cause her to burst into tears. Even a friendly question like "What's new?" upset her. Because she couldn't talk about what had happened, conversations became stilted. Cheryl really didn't understand that her own silence contributed to the distance she felt. Although everyone said that they didn't blame her for what happened, she blamed herself, so she could only assume that her failure to protect her sister was the reason for their detachment.

She found herself staying at home more and just watching TV. She spent many sleepless nights soothed by midnight snacks and many daytime hours in front of mind-numbing TV shows with bags of potato chips, bowls of corn chips, gallons of ice cream, and oooh, those Snickers bars. By the time she started paying any attention to school again, she'd gained thirty pounds and had nearly failing grades. But she really didn't care. Nothing was all that important.

Although very bright, she just couldn't get interested in school during her entire senior year. Her friends encouraged her to try, but they finally gave up. After reducing her impressive academic record into a mediocre high-school career, she graduated weighing almost two hundred pounds. She still had a pretty face, but it was buried in her chubby cheeks, and her once lustrous, thick, light brown hair became dull and limp through lack of care. Her sparkling blue eyes lost their glint and turned the bluish gray of an ocean on an overcast day. Cheryl did go out on the occasional date, but as her girth grew and her wardrobe shrank, she stopped going out altogether, figuring that nobody would want her anyway. Why bother?

After graduation, she looked around for a job. Her lack of employable skills led her to an entry-level job at Wal-Mart. She really didn't need to work, since she still lived at home. Her dad had died prematurely at age forty from diabetes and heart disease, but he had made certain that they were well provided for financially.

Cheryl, only seven, had been devastated at the time, but her mom, Charlotte, had done a reasonably good job filling the void. But now Cheryl was spending most of her time taking care of her widowed mother.

Unfortunately, Charlotte had smoked two packs a day for about forty years and was in and out of the hospital with obstructive lung disease and heart failure. She was tied to an oxygen tank. Although her legs were capable of walking, her lungs wouldn't permit it. It was only four or five years after Joy's death that Charlotte had become disabled. Mostly, her mother was tied to a wheelchair, and Cheryl was tied to her. Charlotte ate next to nothing, and as a result, Cheryl never really learned how to cook. So she ate mostly junk food, fast food, and the occasional "gourmet" TV dinner.

Charlotte's disability had an odd effect on Cheryl. Rather than bemoaning her fate, burdened by her mother's dependency, she became empowered by it. Taking on more responsibility at home had spurred her to do more with her own life. Once deciding to become a dental assistant, she flew through the coarse work with ease, finishing at the top of her class. Cheryl landed her first job without effort and was very happy doing something more useful than manning a cash register at Wal-Mart.

*　　　　　　*　　　　　　*

While at Friday's, Cheryl's mood gradually improved throughout the evening. She always had a good time with the girls—Wendy, Susan, Carol, and Teresa. Their friendship, forged in high school, was still as strong as ever, which was a testament to Cheryl's own worth. No matter how much she had rebuffed them during difficult times, they remained true. Cheryl's good-natured, easygoing attitude and sense of humor always made for pleasant company, even when she wasn't at her best. Though she was no longer the life of the party or a fashion plate, she was still their best friend.

By the time Cheryl returned home, she had a smile on her face. She wasn't surprised to find her mother asleep in the wheelchair in front of the TV, snoring loudly. Cheryl wheeled her into the bedroom and helped her into bed. She gathered pillows to prop her up, but as soon as Charlotte lay down, a coughing fit ensued. Cheryl hated feeling so utterly helpless. Her mother would turn several different colors, none of which seemed humanly possible, before settling back down to a very pale white with tinges of blue. Cheryl was happy that at least she had never started smoking. *Okay*, she thought to herself. *I may be addicted to Snickers, but that's a helluva lot better than cigarettes. At least Snickers can't kill me.*

Having settled her mother in, Cheryl began her nightly routine. As she put on her nightshirt, she avoided the mirror at all costs, hating to look at her naked body. Once between the sheets, she couldn't help thinking about her breakdown earlier in the day. Why had she been so upset? She couldn't really come up with an answer, but the unpleasant memory of her reflection prompted her to consider giving dieting one more try. But the very idea of giving up her Snickers bars made her anxious. In an effort to let those thoughts go, she concentrated on her mother's wheezy breathing in the next room and fell asleep.

Just as Cheryl was leaving the house for work the next morning, her mother had another one of her coughing fits, which delayed her. When her mom was finally okay, Cheryl talked with their neighbor, Mrs. Curtis, to make sure the woman would check in on her mother a little earlier than usual. Her mom and Mrs. Curtis usually had coffee together each morning and played a few games of gin rummy, but Cheryl was a little more worried about Charlotte today and didn't want too much time to pass before someone checked on her. Her mom wore one of those panic buttons around her neck in case of emergency, but Cheryl couldn't be too careful.

All of this made Cheryl late for work. As she entered the first procedure room, her boss, Dr. Weiner, glanced up at her with a brief but stony stare.

"Good afternoon," he said sarcastically.

Cheryl quickly took Janie's place on the stool opposite him, almost knocking over the instrument table in the process. The new girl, Janie, was actually quite slim, so the setup hadn't allowed for Cheryl's girth. Cheryl saw the look Dr. Weiner gave her and tried to ignore it. He had warned her just last week, after a similar incident, that if she continued to put on weight, she might be out of a job. He had pointed out to her that he was unable to enlarge his procedure rooms to accommodate her 230-pound body.

"Adjust the light please, Cheryl," he said tersely.

"Better?" Cheryl asked. Dr. Weiner nodded. She picked up the suction rod, anticipating her boss's needs every step of the way, handing him just the right instrument before he asked. She was good and didn't want to be fired. She wanted to make him feel that she was indispensable, fat or thin.

Hours later, the office receptionist, Tina, stuck her head into each of the procedure rooms. "I'm going to the deli—anyone want anything?" Cheryl ordered a tossed salad. Tina looked at her strangely. "Is that all you want? Who are you kidding?"

Cheryl was thinking about maybe starting her diet, but looked at Tina and said, "Yeah, you're right. Just kidding. Get me a corned beef special with a side of potato salad, and a large Pepsi."

Later, as the two women ate their lunches in the all-purpose room, Tina looked at Cheryl quizzically across the table.

"Are you thinking about going on a diet again?"

"I don't know. One minute I think I should, and then the next minute I think it's pointless. I've dieted so many times in the past, and I lose some weight, but then I just put it all back on again and then some. Ugh, it's so frustrating! But I don't know … maybe this time it could be different. I was thinking of going to my doctor and getting some diet pills. Maybe if I could just get a jump start, I could do better. It's just so hard, and I'm really not up for failing again."

"I have a friend who went on that South Beach Diet, and she's doing really well. She's lost over thirty pounds already," Tina interjected.

"I'm not sure I can face another supposed miracle diet." Cheryl said forlornly. "I really hate being fat … but I love eating. I'm just not sure I can do it, you know?"

"I know this guy … he's a waiter, around food all the time. He used to be really big. About two years ago, he lost over a hundred pounds and started playing ice hockey again. Now he plays three and four times a week, he looks fabulous."

"How did he do it? Do you know?" Cheryl asked, anticipating a diet she'd already tried—and failed.

"Well, I asked him, and he told me he owed everything to his family doctor. I asked him if his doctor had prescribed some pills or something, and he laughed. He said, 'She didn't give me a prescription. She gave me a new attitude.' I really wasn't sure what he was talking about, but maybe I could get his doctor's name for you, if you're interested."

"That might be an idea. God knows I don't have anything better to try." Cheryl polished off her drippy corned-beef special, licking the mayonnaise-like sauce from her fingers as she contemplated seeing this doctor. Of course, Cheryl already knew that attitude wouldn't be enough, but maybe the woman would be willing to provide medication to help her succeed.

Chapter Two

April 2005

Today, Cheryl finally had her first doctor's appointment with the new family doctor that Tina had recommended. She was both eager and apprehensive—eager to get started on a new diet, and apprehensive about what the doctor might find.

Locating the office had not been easy. Although it was only four or five blocks from work, she'd walked by it twice. It was on the lower level of a town house, with the entryway below eye level, half a flight down from the sidewalk.

The waiting room, when she found it, was very welcoming. The comfortable-looking chairs and prints on the wall gave it an atmosphere more like a living room than an office, and the scattered magazines seemed to add a lived-in feeling.

Two women sat at the front desk. The one Cheryl dealt with was very professional, but seemed a little standoffish. Or perhaps Cheryl was projecting her own discomfort. The woman asked her for her insurance card and co-pay, then gave her a bunch of papers on a clipboard to complete—all without a smile, but admittedly she was quite busy.

Cheryl took a seat and began completing the forms. Other patients came and went; the more she waited, the more anxious she became. Her mind drifted, wondering if she was doing the right thing.

She was brought out of her trance by a voice calling her name.

"Could you please follow me," said the small black woman as she led Cheryl from the waiting room into a long, carpeted hall opening up into several exam rooms. "Please step on the scale." Cheryl really didn't want to, but she did.

"Do I have to look?" she managed to blurt out, embarrassed and ashamed at what she knew wouldn't be a pretty number.

"No, that's fine. I'll just record it for the doctor." Cheryl really didn't want to look, but in the end, she opened her eyes just enough to steal a peek. *Egads—235.* She had gained another five pounds since scheduling the appointment. She knew that she had really been overindulging. Ever since deciding to try dieting again, she had been on a relentless mission to consume all her favorite foods before putting herself in diet prison. This was sort of like the condemned man's last meal, she had told herself—only her last meal had lasted about two months.

She wished she hadn't had to wait so long for the appointment. First, she had had to change her primary-care physician through her HMO; she could only do that on the first of the month. Then, it was recommended that she schedule a physical because she was a new patient. She had to wait another month before she could be seen. She hoped she liked this doctor after all she'd been through.

The exam room was small, but fortunately, not overly clinical. One wall was a burned orange color with a Picasso print of similar hues hanging in the middle. The exam table cover was a royal blue, picking up the small slashes of blue contained in the print. A large brochure holder hung on the opposite wall, displaying pamphlets for what seemed like every disease known to mankind. Then again, Cheryl didn't spot any brochures on dieting.

Cheryl sat nervously, waiting for the doctor. As if hospital gowns weren't embarrassing enough, the one they had given her was too small. Or, she realized with a wince, maybe she was too large. She was already sweating, despite the cool breeze provided by air-conditioning. Her discomfort compounded when the medical assistant had to go in search of a larger blood pressure cuff because her arm was too big for the regular one. At least her blood pressure was 130/85—not as high it was the last time she had gone to the doctor six months ago. Her previous doctor had told her that it was borderline, but hadn't put her on any medication. She had breathed a sigh of relief at the time; she hated to take pills. He had just told her to decrease the salt in her diet and try to lose some weight. *Yeah,* she thought, *that really worked well.*

The doctor suddenly appeared with a knock on the door. "Good morning— I'm Nikki Lang," she said, extending her hand to offer a firm grip.

Cheryl was nonplussed. The doctor standing before her wore jeans and Docksider loafers. She did have a white coat and a name tag, but she didn't exactly look like a doctor. Her hair was long and streaked with gray. Cheryl really couldn't tell how old she was.

Cheryl's hoped the doctor hadn't noticed the sweat on her palm.

"I see you're here for a routine physical. Are there any particular problems you wanted to discuss?" Dr. Lang settled down on a stool and flipped through Cheryl's medical chart, reviewing the history form Cheryl had completed while in the waiting room. Cheryl had been pretty healthy, so her medical history was actually rather boring.

Finally, Cheryl got up the nerve to speak. "I wanted to know if I could get some diet pills or something. A co-worker of mine told me about a patient of yours who had done really well with your help—plays ice hockey all the time now—and I wanted to know if you could do the same with me. You know, put me on a diet."

"I don't believe in diets," was the doctor's reply as she looked up at Cheryl.

The abruptness of the comment stunned Cheryl. Tears welled in Cheryl's eyes. Finding a suitable diet had been the whole point of this visit. She had finally gotten up enough courage to ask about pills, only to be shot down. She had half a mind to walk right out of the office and demand her $20 co-pay back. The only thing that stopped her was the fact that she was buck naked under a thin hospital gown.

"If you go on a diet, you'll go off a diet, so what's the point?" Dr. Lang continued. "What you have to do is change your eating habits."

By this time, Cheryl was hardly listening to anything Dr. Lang was saying; she was so angry that she had wasted her morning.

"If you're really interested in losing some weight, I'm willing to help you," Dr. Lang continued. "But you need to be willing to work at it."

The tears began trickling down Cheryl's cheeks.

Dr. Lang handed her some tissues without pausing. "I'm sure you've been on diets before. Did they work?'

"Well," Cheryl sniffed, "the one diet that really worked well for me was the Atkins Diet. I lost nearly fifty pounds!"

"But it didn't work, did it?"

"What do you mean? I lost fifty pounds."

"So, how much did you weigh after that?"

"One hundred and seventy pounds."

"And how much do you weigh now?"

"Two hundred and thirty-five."

"Look … Cheryl," Dr. Lang said after quickly checking her name on the chart. "I can tell that you really want to lose some weight. And I'll do what I can to help you. I truly wish there was a magic pill I could give you or a failsafe program I could recommend. But there isn't. Take the Atkins Diet: you lost the weight, but then gained it all back … and then some. So I ask you again: did the diet work?"

Cheryl began to get the doctor's point. Yes, she had lost weight. But not only had she put the fifty pounds back on after stopping, she had even added another ten.

"I guess it really didn't."

"Exactly," Dr. Lang said more sympathetically. "Diets don't work. You have to change your eating habits, and changing habits takes a long time. What's a habit anyway?"

"I guess it's something you do that's not good, like smoking."

"Well, yes, that's a bad habit. But what's a good habit?"

"I don't know." Cheryl thought she was beginning to understand. "Maybe like not eating junk food?"

"Yes, that would be a good habit. So is turning off a light when you walk out of the room, or saying 'thank you' when someone does something nice for you. So, I'll ask again. What's a habit?'

"Something you do all the time?"

"Exactly! Something you do without thinking." Cheryl felt like a student being grilled by her teacher. But at that moment, Dr. Lang smiled, dispelling that impression.

"Yes," Dr. Lang continued, nodding, "it happens almost automatically without effort. So how long do you think it takes to establish a habit—or, for that matter, get rid of a bad habit?"

"I dunno … a few weeks, maybe?"

"I see here on your history sheet that your mother suffers from lung disease and heart failure. Is she a smoker?"

Cheryl nodded in the affirmative.

"Do you think if she stopped smoking for three or four weeks, she would have licked the habit?"

Cheryl shook her head.

"You're right. Habits take anywhere from six to nine months to make or break—some maybe less time, some more. The point that I'm making is that changing your eating habits takes a lot longer than a few weeks. If you go on a diet for a few weeks or even a few months, how much headway have you made in changing your eating habits?"

Cheryl felt as if she were beginning to comprehend what the doctor was saying. But at the same time, her sense of hopelessness had not lifted. She knew that she just didn't have the willpower or the patience to do something for nine whole months.

"It's not just all the individual foods you eat," the doctor went on. "It's how you shop, what you keep in the house, how you store food, how often you eat out, how many times a day you eat, or if you eat when you're angry or sad. The list goes on and on."

Cheryl was really wondering why she'd bothered coming here. She had thought that this doctor was going to have some new way to help her lose weight. Now, she was feeling even more frustrated than before. The task seemed more daunting than ever.

Suddenly, the doctor paused and looked up at Cheryl in a way that made her feel exposed by more than just her ill-fitting gown—as if her thoughts were an open book. It somehow didn't surprise Cheryl when Dr. Lang abruptly changed gears. .

"Cheryl, I see that you're a dental assistant. I presume that you brush your teeth every morning and night?"

"Of course, but I don't see your point," she said through gritted teeth, beginning to get angry.

"Did you always brush your teeth regularly, even though your mother had told you to?"

Cheryl remembered letting herself go after Joy died. She'd stopped doing her hair and her makeup. Half the time, she hadn't bothered getting dressed. What was the point? She had even stopped brushing her teeth. As a matter of fact, she'd gotten the idea of becoming a dental assistant when she'd gotten several painful cavities fixed. It was all that junk food, she knew. The cavities had reminded her that it wasn't all about appearances. Brushing was a good idea. By the time she was taking dental tech classes, she was flossing regularly.

Returning to the doctor's question, Cheryl shook her head as her anger faded.

"Do you find it a great effort to brush your teeth every day?"

"No, in fact, I even floss every day."

"So that's precisely what I'm talking about. Once you establish a new habit, it sticks, and you don't have to think about it anymore. That's what you have to do with eating habits. Do it slowly, only addressing a couple habits at a time." Dr. Lang took a breath and continued. "The real problem, I find, is that you have to know which important habits to establish first as you work toward your goal. It's really amazing to me that so many people go about the very important job of learning to eat healthily with so little knowledge. How proficient would you be as a dental assistant if you'd read one book on dental care and then tried to be good at your job?"

"Not so good."

"Learning to eat right for your health might be one of the most important jobs in your life. Don't you think it might be worthwhile to educate yourself about doing it right?"

Cheryl nodded in agreement. But she still wasn't really sure she could do it.

"Look, Cheryl, let's start with one habit. What fluids do you drink during the day?"

"Black coffee with two sugars, Pepsi, and fruit juice."

"How many fruit juices, and how many Pepsis?'

"Two or three."

"Of each or both?"

"Probably three combined a day."

"Do you have any idea how many calories that represents?"

"A hundred or two?"

"Minimally, 450 calories, and that depends on what fruit juice and how many ounces. If it's one of those sixteen-ounce bottles, then it's more than 550 calories. Take a guess at how many pounds that represents in one year."

"I dunno … ten, maybe?"

"If you changed nothing else in your diet, but stopped drinking your calories, you could lose anywhere from forty-five to fifty-five pounds in one year!"

"Really? But what do I drink?"

"Diet drinks."

"But they taste terrible; I can't stand them."

"Look, Cheryl: here are a couple of pages that I'm writing on the topic of acquired taste from my diet book—or, should I say, healthy eating book. Why don't you read them, and when you come back in a month, we'll talk about it again. As a matter of fact, you might want to pick up the other two of the first three chapters of the book at the front desk, which will review what we've already discussed today."

Dr. Lang finished taking Cheryl's history, then did the physical. When she was finished, she told Cheryl to schedule her next appointment, so they could review her lab work at that time and continue their discussion.

The pleasant medical assistant returned to take Cheryl's blood and give her a tetanus shot that was due.

Cheryl left the office unsure of how she felt. She wasn't angry anymore, but she also wasn't very happy. She had thought that she would walk out of the office with a pill in hand ready to change her life, and instead she was actually a bit disheartened. As she walked to the deli to meet Teresa for lunch, she thought about all that Dr. Lang had told her.

*   *   *

Teresa managed a retail shoe store on South Street, so she was able to skip out for forty-five minutes for lunch. When Cheryl met her at the deli, Teresa was full of questions about the doctor visit.

"It didn't go so well," Cheryl responded. "I thought I'd get some great diet, but all she talked about was changing habits—how hard it is, how long it takes, and how much knowledge is required to eat right. Basically, I think it was a great big flop."

"Didn't she ask you to do anything at all?"

"Well, she said I should drink diet instead of regular soda and fruit juice and put Splenda in my coffee. She said I could lose up to forty-five or fifty-five pounds in a year even if I did nothing else."

"Wow, forty-five or fifty-five pounds. You know, I drink diet soda."

"Yeah, but you like it. I hate it. It's disgusting!"

"Cheryl, you look like you're about to burst into tears. Was it really that bad?"

"Oh, Teresa, I'm just so frustrated. I really had my hopes up. I wanted to do it this time, but it just seems so … impossible. You know how hard I've tried in the past, but nothing ever seems to really work." Tears started trickling down Cheryl's cheeks yet again.

Teresa grabbed her friend's hand and squeezed it. "Is there anything I can do?"

"What can you do? I mean, geez, it's up to me, isn't it?"

"Well, I dunno. Maybe there's something I can help with. Tell me what else the doctor talked about. Maybe I can learn something."

"You're thin. What do you need to learn?"

"Maybe about how not to get fat. You've seen my mother. Is that what I have to look forward to?"

Cheryl smiled. She couldn't imagine Teresa looking like her mom, who was nearly as large as Cheryl, but had bony knees and small boobs. Teresa smiled with her. "You know, my mother was once my size. I really don't want to become my mother, so help me out here."

Cheryl dried her tears and recounted what she had learned. "She said I need to start by changing just a few small habits at a time, not to actually go on a diet. That it takes a while to establish habits, but once you do, they stick. She used my daily flossing as an example."

Teresa looked at her watch. Their food still hadn't arrived. "If our food doesn't come soon, I'm going to have to take mine with me back to the shop."

"Yeah, you and me both!"

"Getting back to what the doctor said … does it make any sense to you?"

"It all makes sense," Cheryl replied. "It's just that … that … I dunno."

"It's just what, Cheryl?" Teresa prodded.

"It just seems like it will take forever. I mean, nine months to establish one stinky habit?"

"Yeah, but remember what the doctor said about you and flossing. Once you learn a habit, it sticks. God knows you certainly bug me about it enough!"

Cheryl grinned. She could be really annoying about getting other people to floss. "I know, but it just seems like it will take eons to lose any weight."

"What have you got to lose? Why not at least try? If you don't try, you're still going to be the same size a year from now."

"I'll think about it," she said, not very convincingly. "Oh, look our food is finally coming."

Just as their food arrived, Cheryl noticed a few of the papers that Dr. Lang had given her sticking out of her purse. "I almost forgot these," she said as she extricated the papers from her purse's innards. "Dr. Lang gave me some chapters from the book she's writing. These are the first few on habits ... and something about taste." She looked at the title. "'Acquired Taste'—that's it. Maybe you'd like to read them?" She handed the pages to Teresa.

Teresa laid them down next to her plate and started reading while she ravenously took large bites of her sandwich. As she finished each page, she handed it back to Cheryl. Having nothing better to do, Cheryl read them too.

After finishing the short chapters, Teresa said, "Well, it kinda makes sense, don't you think? I used to hate beer, but when I went to those wild frat parties on Penn Campus, I didn't want to feel like a real loser, so I drank it anyway, and now I really like it. What about you?"

"Ugh, I can't stand beer—never could. It tastes terrible."

"Isn't there anything that you eat or drink now that you didn't like when you were younger?"

"No."

Teresa sighed.

Cheryl could tell her friend was really frustrated with her. But Teresa didn't understand. How could she? She'd never been overweight or even on a diet. She was as slim as she was in high school—and with her thick, dark hair and perfect skin, she was a guy magnet. How could she possible know how Cheryl felt?

Cheryl was happy when Teresa changed the subject. She didn't want to talk about it anymore.

They finished their lunch with some momentary idle chatter about Wendy's upcoming wedding. Cheryl told Teresa she would stop by her store at the end of the day, to find the new pair of shoes Cheryl had promised herself, and then they both went back to work.

Before moving on with our story, let's review the important points that Cheryl has learned thus far.

STEP 1: HOW TO GET STARTED
Stop Drinking Your Calories
By
Nikki Lang, MD

Calories that you drink do absolutely nothing toward satisfying your appetite. If, for example, you drink a soda with your meal, do you eat less food than if you hadn't had the soda? The answer, of course, is no. You're still going to eat the same amount. Your meal then contains an additional 150 calories. If you do this at lunch and dinner every day, you are consuming an additional 300 calories without any further appetite satisfaction. You may be thinking, "But I like soda." Over the next several chapters, we will discuss how your present likes and dislikes will factor into this plan, but for the moment, let's put this thought on hold.

So here you are, drinking an extra 300 calories (in soda, fruit juice, or milk) without any further appetite suppression. Let's review what that means in pounds. Since there are 365 days in a year, and there are 3,600 calories in one pound, then 10 calories a day times 365 equals 3,650 calories, or approximately 1 pound. Every additional 100 calories ingested per day for one year represents 10 pounds; therefore, an additional 300 calories daily equals 30 pounds in one year. (300 calories x 365 days in a year = 109,500 calories. 109,500 ÷ 3,600 calories = 30.42 pounds in a year.) Mind-boggling, isn't it? For every 100 calories less per day ingested, you could lose as much as 10 whole pounds per year.

Very small changes over time can make huge differences.

So let's address other things you might drink on any given day—coffee or tea, for example. If you drink your coffee or tea black, then you are drinking nothing more than flavored water (with regard to calories), so there are no calories to consider. However, if you use cream, sugar, or both, then you must count those calories. As an example, if you use 2 rounded teaspoons of sugar in 2 cups of coffee or tea per day, you have 2 tablespoons of sugar each day (3 flat teaspoons = 1 tablespoon). Each table-spoon of sugar contains 45 calories, which means that the 2 tablespoons of sugar equals 90 calories per day—or 9 pounds per year. By eliminating 2 sodas and 2 tablespoons of sugar (using artificial sweetener instead) each day, you could lose 39 pounds in one year.

Very small changes do add up!

Another interesting way to really appreciate small incremental changes is to create a warehouse in your mind that is going to house all the food you won't eat for the next year. So, if you were to visit the part of your warehouse that housed the soda (or juice) that you didn't drink in one year, at 2 sodas a day, it would presently contain 61 *cases* of soda. The shelf holding the sugar, if you abstained from 2 tablespoons a day, would have approximately 5 five-pound bags of sugar, and 1 two-pound bag of sugar. We will revisit this warehouse concept in the future, just to drive home the importance of small changes.

So Step 1 in this journey to eat better and be slimmer is to stop drinking your calories. We won't address alcohol consumption at this point, except to say that fewer calories are better, light beer is superior to regular beer, and less is always an improvement.

ACQUIRED TASTE
What Is It, and How Does It Work?
By
Nikki Lang, MD

"Acquired taste" refers to the concept of learning to like something that you've never liked before. One of the simplest illustrations is that of the beer drinker. I'd be willing to bet that very few people liked beer the first time they tasted it … and yet today, millions of people love beer. Are they forcing themselves to drink it? Obviously not. They have learned to savor the taste in spite of their initial aversion. Why did they acquire a taste for beer? Well, maybe when they were younger, they thought it was cool. Or perhaps they just wanted to fit in with their peers. Or, although they didn't particularly like the taste, they liked how it made them feel—they liked the buzz. Whatever the reason, they chose to drink beer, and by repeating the experience over and over, they learned to like what they initially thought was awful. They are no longer forcing themselves to drink it; they truly enjoy it, want it, and think it tastes great. How does this happen?

Earlier, I mentioned that we human beings are not terribly fond of change and find it very difficult. Well, that "shortcoming" can also be an asset, depending on how we approach it. We love and crave what is familiar to us.

Anything that we do every day becomes desirable, comforting, or relaxing. Whether it's taking off our tie or shoes at the end of a day, having our first cup of coffee in the morning, or engaging in grooming rituals like brushing our teeth or washing our hair, sameness breeds comfort.

Do you remember how much fun you had on your last vacation, but also how good it felt to be home in familiar surroundings? Well, the only way that something can become familiar and comfortable is through repeated exposure. The more we experience a particular activity, or food, or environment, the more comfortable it becomes, and generally the more we like it.

Acquired taste requires a great deal of repetition.

If you want to drink water or diet drinks instead of regular soda or juice, you need to learn to like water or diet drinks—or both.

Now, a few little tricks can ease the process. Our palates—that is to say, our taste buds—are also reluctant to change, so it's often necessary to blindside them. Say you are a Pepsi drinker who has tried Diet Pepsi in the past and thought it was awful. Since your palate was expecting regular Pepsi, it reacted to the unfamiliar taste: "Yuck!" Similarly, just think how awful vodka or gin would taste if you were expecting natural spring water—double yuck! Expectation plays a very important role in how good something tastes.

To avoid that issue when switching to diet drinks, pick a flavor of soda that you rarely drink. Your taste buds will not hold a preconception of what it's supposed to taste like. It may not taste great, but it will taste okay.

Continue to drink these other diet-flavored drinks for several months, and avoid all cola for at least three months. If you basically have a preference for cola, after a three-month hiatus, Diet Pepsi will taste pretty good. Continue to drink Diet Pepsi for the next three to four months (without ever drinking a regular Pepsi), and you will find by that time a regular Pepsi will not taste particularly good—in fact, it may actually taste too sweet!

You have now acquired a taste for diet soda. It has become your preference, and it actually tastes better to you than a regular Pepsi. Don't believe me? Ask other diet-soda drinkers. Better yet, put this book down for the next several months and begin the experiment. Many of my patients over the years have reported back to me after our discussions that it was easier than they had expected to acquire a taste for new foods and drinks. Many who had already learned to drink diet soda, but had not yet applied the concept to food, agreed that they no longer even enjoyed regular soda.

Perhaps you too can begin to benefit from acquired taste. Stop digging in your heels and avoiding change. You have to open up to the idea that changing your taste buds may not be as difficult as it first seems—and it's crucial to your future success.

ON ESTABLISHING HABITS
By
Nikki Lang, MD

The dictionary defines "habit" as "a recurrent, often unconscious pattern of behavior that is acquired through frequent repetition." Once you have acquired a taste for diet soda, you'll have developed a good habit. Obviously, the concepts of habit and acquired taste overlap, but it is important to make some distinction. As Cheryl learned, many different habits (what, where, how, and when) are involved in eating.

So what do you do? How do you successfully change your eating habits? The simple answer, which I'm sure you've already figured out, is to address only a few habits at a time. Trying to change hundreds of habits simultaneously, as you do when you go on a diet, is totally unrealistic. The chances of success are minimal. So why not give yourself a fighting chance by gradually changing just a few habits at a time, instead of all of them all at once?

So, if your choice of beverages (Step 1) is the only habit that you try to change initially, you'll still lose weight. By doing just this simple step, you will also learn the very important concept of acquired taste. You will learn what establishing a good habit is all about—and that, if you are patient and take it one step at a time, changing habits isn't nearly as difficult as it first seems.

I don't want to leave this discussion of habits just yet; some important aspects of habit changing still need to be reviewed.

Establishing a new habit, as we have said, requires repetition. The more often you do something, and the longer you do it, the sooner it will become an unconscious behavior. The good news: even if you don't do it every single time without fail, you can still be well on the road to establishing that habit. The bad news: the more frequently you don't do it, the longer it's going to take.

Pavlov proved that dogs could learn to salivate at the ringing of a bell, once they had associated that bell with dinner. Sometime later Skinner came along and established the concept of intermittent reinforcement. Let me give you an example. He put a mouse in a cage with a simple lever that dispensed food. Every time the mouse stepped on the lever, it received a food pellet. After a while, he stopped giving the mouse any food. The mouse would continue to push on the lever, but after a relatively short time, when it consistently received nothing in return, it stopped stepping on the lever. Next, he did the same experiment, but instead of giving food every time the mouse stepped on the lever, he gave it food every third or fourth time. When he stopped giving the mouse food entirely, the behavior persisted far longer.

It works precisely the same way with negative reinforcement. If he had given the mouse small electric shocks every time it stepped on a certain grid of the cage, the mouse would have learned to avoid that grid much more quickly than if he only shocked the mouse every third or fourth time.

Let's apply this to humans. Let's say that you develop significant heartburn every time you have a cup of coffee. How long do you think it would take for you to stop drinking coffee? How much longer do you think it would take for you to stop if you only developed heartburn every third or fourth time you drank it?

So how does this apply to developing good eating habits? If, as I advise, you were to begin drinking diet sodas, but every fourth time you gave in to temptation and drank a regular soda, then a real habit change would take much longer. Likewise, if I were to advise you to eat breakfast every morning, and you were to only eat it some mornings, how much longer do you think it will take to establish that behavior as a habit?

The good news is, however, that it will still become a habit; all is not lost if you occasionally slip up. Just get back into the routine as soon as possible.

Remember, the repetition of any behavior adds up to change!

Let's continue with our story and find out how Cheryl deals with change.

Chapter Three

April 2005

"Mom, I'm home," Cheryl called from the foyer. She was a little early. Dr. Weiner's last patient had cancelled, so she'd managed to get out sooner than usual. She had stopped by KFC and picked up a bucket of chicken for dinner. The mail was still on the floor from that day's delivery. She picked it up and idly went through it as she made her way to the kitchen to drop off the chicken. An envelope from that new doctor was in the mail. It had been three weeks since she had visited Dr. Lang, but she still hadn't done a thing. She mostly tried to forget about the entire visit. She had an appointment next week, but she wasn't sure she was going to keep it. She put the envelope down unopened; she really didn't want to know what was in it. She went back out into the living room to check on her mom, who was nearing the end of her weekly bridge game. She could barely make out their conversation.

Although their house was semidetached—connected to another home on one side—it was actually quite large. Besides the large entryway, it originally had had a large study on the first floor, along with the separate dining room, living room, and kitchen. When she was really little, Cheryl's family had built an extension on the back, adding a master bedroom and bath. When Cheryl's mother had become ill so many years ago, Cheryl had moved down from the second floor to be near her mother. The den had become Cheryl's bedroom, and the second floor was rarely used.

"Mom ... Mom, where is it? I smell it. Mrs. Curtis, why do you let her do that?"

"Oh, come on, Cheryl. Your mother has so few pleasures in life. Why deprive her of smoking now?"

"You know why—you especially, Mrs. O'Hara. Didn't your husband once work for the fire department? She's got oxygen. What are you women trying to do, burn us down? Where is it?" Cheryl finally spied the small ashtray shoved under her mother's wheelchair, still containing smoldering cigarette ashes. "Who buys these things for you?" she asked as she bent over to give her mother a kiss on the forehead. "I love you, but honestly, one of these days you're going to go up in flames. Really, Mom, where'd you get these?" She glared at her mother's three cohorts in crime. They all smiled like little girls caught with their hands in the cookie jar.

"Seriously," Cheryl continued, her anger building, "you all know how danger-ous it is to smoke near oxygen. If you feel compelled to give her a cigarette, then for God's sake, please take away the oxygen. Then you can watch her cough and turn all those ugly colors. Maybe after seeing that, you won't give her the ciga-rettes." The women looked a bit chastened, but she wasn't really sure they were listening to her. *Why is it,* Cheryl wondered, *that as people age, they become more like children?*

They had finished their last hand and were adding up the score to see who had won when the phone rang. It was Teresa. "You have any plans for tonight?"

"Not really, but I don't want to leave my mom alone. She had her bridge friends over, and someone brought her cigarettes. I won't feel comfortable until I make sure there aren't any more in the house."

"Well, why don't you see what you can sort out? Carol's husband is out of town this weekend, so we all decided to go over there for a girls' night in. Thought we'd rent an old movie, get drunk, and pig out. You up for it?"

"How do we get drunk at Carol's house? Isn't she still in recovery?"

"Of course, Just kidding. You game? We thought we'd meet around eight or eight thirty."

"Sounds good to me, if I can get Mom sorted out. I'll call you if I can't."

Cheryl wheeled her mother into the dining room to have some dinner with her and tell her about her day. She set the table and chattered about some of the patients she had seen earlier, then asked her mom about her bridge game and who won.

"Maggie and Anna always seem to win. I think they cheat," Charlotte said cau-tiously, obviously still expecting to be chastised further about the cigarettes.

Cheryl placed a plate of food in front of Charlotte, then sat down with her own and dived in. She was starving, and fried chicken was one of her favorites. Her mom mostly pushed the food around her plate.

"What's the matter? Don't you like it? It's really good."

"I'm just not that hungry. I ate a lot for lunch."

"So what did you have?"

"I had a tuna fish sandwich and some potato salad. I even had some ice cream for dessert. So what are your plans for tonight?"

"Well, Carol's husband is out of town this week, and Teresa called. They're having a girls' night in. I was thinking of going, but I'm afraid that you may have more cigarettes in the house, so I'm thinking of staying home to keep an eye on you."

Cheryl knew just what buttons to push. She knew her mother didn't want to be responsible for keeping her home. Charlotte reached into her skirt pocket and handed the remains of a soft pack of Marlboros to her daughter.

Cheryl just stared at her without saying another word. Out came two more single cigarettes.

"That's it, I promise."

"Are you sure? Mom, I do love you, and I just want to keep you around a little longer. Do you understand that?"

"Come 'ere, give me a big hug. I know you care, sweetheart. It's just so hard. Maggie was right today. I really don't have many pleasures in life, and cigarettes just happen to be one of them. Just think how you'd feel if I went around stealing your stash of Snickers bars and stopped you dead in your tracks every time you bit into one."

"But Snickers won't kill me, Ma!"

"Are you sure?" Charlotte raised one eyebrow and stared at her daughter until Cheryl looked away.

"Thanks for giving me the cigarettes, Mom. I really appreciate it."

While Cheryl was cleaning up after dinner, she noticed about three quarters of an unfinished tuna fish sandwich lurking under a Styrofoam container in the garbage can. So much for the "big lunch" her mother had had. If the smoking didn't kill her, she'd die of starvation.

Her mom had been very pretty in her day; Cheryl had seen pictures of her. But from memory, it seemed as if she'd always looked the same, with cropped gray hair and wizened, crêpe-like, blue-tinged skin draped over her prominent bones. Charlotte didn't appear to have an ounce of fat on her. She'd almost be scary looking if she didn't have the kindest, warmest eyes in the world. Everyone who knew her loved her. Make no mistake about it: she could be stubborn, but she didn't have an evil cell in her body. *If only I could give Mom some of my own fat,* Cheryl mused. *Wouldn't that be the perfect solution?*

Cheryl changed her clothes and checked up on her mom, who was settled in front of the TV. Charlotte was able to get around when she had to, so Cheryl knew she'd be all right.

She glanced at the unopened envelope from the doctor. She decided it could wait, then dashed out the door to Carol's.

When Cheryl arrived, everyone was already ensconced in the living room— shoes off, legs propped up, munching on popcorn and waiting for Cheryl. They were ready to start their chosen movie, *First Wives Club.*

"Sorry I'm a little late, guys—had some trouble finding a parking spot."

"No problem," said Wendy. "Get your fat ass over here and make yourself comfy."

"That popcorn smells really good." And with that, Cheryl plopped down on the couch and grabbed a fistful.

Carol jumped up and asked her what she wanted to drink.

"Pepsi, please."

"I'm really sorry, but I'm all out of Pepsi. I've got Sprite, ginger ale, and orange soda. I've got spring water too, if you want."

"Okay … I'll take a ginger ale, thanks."

When Carol handed Cheryl the ginger ale, everyone was staring at her. Cheryl felt their eyes on her.

"What? Do I have spinach in my teeth or something? What gives?" Judging from their nervous laughter, Cheryl was sure they were up to something, but she hadn't a clue as to what it was.

"No, we were just waiting for you to start the movie," Wendy said.

"Wait no more—your fat-assed highness is here!"

They dimmed the lights a bit and watched the movie. All through the movie, Cheryl had the sense that everyone was staring at her. She did a mental check of her hair and clothes, wondering if she had done something stupid.

Halfway through, Susan piped up. "Pause the movie. I have to pee." Susan was pregnant with child number two, and at seven months along, she found it hard to go longer than an hour or two without a pit stop.

"Anyone want anything else to drink?" Carol asked.

"Another Sprite for me," Wendy answered.

"I'll have some more ginger ale," Cheryl said, starting to get up. "Here let me help you, Carol."

"Not necessary—relax! I'm already up. Anyone else want anything?" No one did.

Carol gave Cheryl her second glass of ginger ale. Cheryl sensed something strange in the air, but whatever it was escaped her. Susan came back from the bathroom, and everyone settled down to watch the end of the movie.

"What a great ending," Cheryl said. "Poetic justice never seems to happen in real life, though."

"Yeah, you're so right. Why do we let men screw with us so easily?" Teresa said. "They always seem to get away with murder, and we're stuck holding the bag."

"And whose fault is that?" Carol asked. "Theirs or ours?"

"Good question," Teresa answered. "Let's leave it at that. This discussion is going to get too philosophical for me. I'm ready for bed." She got up and went to get her coat.

Cheryl got up to follow her out.

"Wait a minute, Cheryl. I need to show you something," Carol said.

By this time, everyone was standing around in the hallway, waiting for Carol to come back out of the kitchen with something hidden under a kitchen towel. She trotted up to Cheryl, who looked at her with a puzzled expression.

With a great flourish, Carol pulled the towel off the bottle of ginger ale. "Tada!"

Cheryl looked at her as if she were nuts. "So … what are you showing me? It's a bottle of ginger ale."

"Look again, dear heart."

Cheryl looked closer and saw the word "diet" in smaller print on the upper part of the label. A smile spread across her face; she knew her friends had put one over on her. Now she knew what had been going on earlier. She should've been mad, but she knew it was because they really cared about her.

"You, my lady, have been drinking diet soda all night. What do you have to say about that?"

"I guess it's not as bad as I thought it was."

Cheryl went home that night feeling good. She felt a little sheepish, but very lucky to have such caring friends.

As Cheryl slipped between the sheets that night, she thought again about how the diet ginger ale really hadn't tasted bad. She suddenly remembered the unread chapter that Dr. Lang had given her. She turned her bedside lamp back on, rummaged around in her night table drawer, and found the forgotten pages.

Upon completion of the chapter, Cheryl turned off the light again, feeling slightly less negative about making changes.

Let's find out what Cheryl learned that made her slightly less resistant to the idea of changing.

WHY IS ACQUIRED TASTE SO IMPORTANT?
By
Nikki Lang, MD

Most people who have a weight problem are fully aware that they don't always eat right. Most people are at least somewhat cognizant of what they should be eating and what they should avoid, but will tell you that they just don't have the discipline to avoid those yummy, comforting, calorie-laden foods that keep beckoning to them.

Constant diligence is probably beyond the ability of most of us, so it is imperative to find a method that doesn't require such vigilance. Once you have acquired a taste for something, like diet soda or water, discipline and vigilance are no longer an issue, because you like the taste. It's what you want, and what you automatically drink without thinking. It has now become a good habit. You no longer need to resist the regular soda, and you no longer feel deprived that you can't have it.

As you apply this concept to more and more healthy foods over time, those good foods will become your preferences, and discipline will become less and less of an issue. **Acquired taste reduces the need for discipline.**

One of the many issues that I have confronted in my medical practice over the years is the narrow range of foods eaten by many obese patients. You might think that they eat anything and everything. Quite the contrary—they often have so many well-ingrained dislikes that it is impossible for them to develop anything even remotely akin to a normal diet. Many of these patients only eat what they ate as a child. Unfortunately, it is mostly fast food or ethnic food that is heavy in starches and fat, almost devoid of vegetables and fruit. These people will never lose weight permanently until they learn to acquire a taste for a greater variety of foods.

In future chapters, we will discuss different ways to fool your palate in an attempt to acquire tastes for new foods.

Chapter Four

April 2005

The next morning, running late as usual, Cheryl spied the envelope from the doctor's office just as she was dashing out the door. She grabbed it and shoved it in her purse. Her workday was predictably hectic, but nothing she couldn't handle. By lunchtime, Cheryl was starving. She'd skipped breakfast as usual—she never seemed to allow enough time for it. But she now had a few extra minutes, so she walked across the street to the deli and ordered a hamburger and cheese fries.

She looked carefully over the glassed refrigeration unit, seeing if she could find a diet drink that she might like. She looked over the fruit-flavored diet Snapples and chose peach. She liked peaches. She took her food back to the office to eat. She tried the Snapple, sipping tentatively at first. It wasn't too bad. It wasn't Pepsi, but it was okay. She could tolerate it.

While she was eating in the all-purpose room, Cheryl spied the envelope sticking out of her purse. She pulled it out, opened it, and found herself staring at her lab results. The list of numbers was accompanied by notations of "normal" and "abnormal." At the bottom was a note that Dr. Lang wanted to review the labs with her during her next visit. Her cholesterol wasn't very good, and her sugar was a bit high. She tried to remember what these numbers had been when she'd last had them tested, but her mind was blank. Was she diabetic? Her father had been diabetic. He had died when he was in his forties from a heart attack; the doctors had blamed diabetes. Geez, was she going to die in her forties? That was too young to die.

Suddenly, Cheryl didn't feel so good. The hamburger and cheese fries she had just eaten settled like lead in her belly, and her heart fluttered as if it would burst through her chest wall. Tina walked in just at that moment. "Cheryl, what's the matter? You look like you've lost your best friend."

"Worse." She extended the lab report to Tina.

Tina looked it over and nonchalantly shrugged. "It doesn't look so bad. Your sugar is just a little high, and so's your cholesterol. It's not the end of the world."

Tina's father was still alive. He hadn't died from diabetes. She didn't know what she was talking about. Could a person be a little bit diabetic? Is that like being a little bit pregnant? Cheryl was terrified. Her father died when she was just seven; she hardly remembered him. She knew nothing about diabetes. She just knew people died from it. She was almost paralyzed from fear. Tina kept talking to her, but Cheryl was listening to her own demons, not to Tina.

"Knock, knock, Cheryl. Are you there?" Finally, Tina tapped her on the shoulder.

Cheryl looked up at Tina and mumbled, "Sorry … I guess I wasn't paying attention."

"Well, I came in here to tell you that Dr. Weiner needs you in room two," Tina told her with an exasperated sigh.

Cheryl nodded in acknowledgement and then slowly moved to room two. She was distracted; she kept offering Dr. Weiner the wrong instruments and failed to adjust the light properly. After the third mishap, Dr. Weiner stopped what he was doing and silently glared at Cheryl.

Cheryl burst into tears and ran out of the office.

Cheryl came back to the office a half hour later and faced Dr. Weiner with slumped shoulders.

"I'm so sorry, Dr. Weiner. I shouldn't have left the office like that. I was really upset about some lab results I received from my doctor's office, but I shouldn't have reacted like that."

"Anything I can do for you?" Dr. Weiner asked "Tina said your cholesterol and your sugar were just a little high. It's really not the end of the world. I'm sure your doctor will sort it out for you."

"You're right," Cheryl agreed, even though she didn't agree at all. Dr. Weiner wasn't diabetic either. What did he know? She knew he was only trying to help, but that didn't make her feel any better.

She left the office that evening feeling really demoralized.

Cheryl walked in the door to her house, looking as if she'd lost three inches in height. She tried to act as if nothing were bothering her, but she knew it was almost impossible to fool her very perceptive mother. At the dinner table, Charlotte finally asked, "What's wrong, Cheryl?"

"Nothing's wrong, Ma. Why do you ask?"

"Honey, I haven't lived with you for thirty-two years without learning something about you. If I say there's something wrong, there's something wrong. Now give!"

Cheryl felt the tears welling up in her eyes again. She turned away and started for the kitchen with the dishes.

"Cheryl Morris, you put those dishes down, and come here, and look me in the eye, and tell me there's nothing wrong!"

Cheryl put down the dishes, walked over to her mother, looked in her eyes, and burst out sobbing. "I think I have diabetes. My sugar is high, and so is my cholesterol and … and … and … Oh, Mom, am I going to die like Daddy?" She knelt down in front of her mother's wheelchair, put her head on Charlotte's lap, and sobbed. Charlotte rubbed her daughter's back and murmured soothing sounds.

Finally, she spoke. "Sweetheart, don't you have an appointment with the doctor next week? Wouldn't it be wise to put all your questions down so that you can ask the doctor when you see her? I don't remember very much about your father's initial diagnosis, but I think the sugar has to be pretty high before they call it diabetes. If I'm not mistaken, a small elevation is just referred to as glucose intolerant, or something like that. You know my sugar was a little high when I was pregnant with you and Joy, but it went back to normal."

Cheryl looked up at her mother, wiping the tears from her cheeks with the back of her hand. "Really?"

"Yes, really."

It had been a long time since Joy's name had been spoken between them. Somehow, the mention of Joy's name put Cheryl's slightly elevated sugar in better perspective.

"You miss her. Don't you, Ma?"

"I do, Cheryl. I miss her a lot."

"Me, too! Oh, Mom, I'm so sorry. I should never have let it happen." Suddenly Cheryl's head was back in her mother's lap. She was crying so hard that her chest was heaving, and she was gasping for breath.

"Oh, honey, it wasn't your fault. You've got to stop blaming yourself. It could just as easily been me who went into the house to answer the phone while looking after Joy. I know that."

Cheryl looked up at her mom, ignoring the tears that were flowing down her cheeks, and stared really hard into her eyes. Charlotte's gaze never left her own.

"You really don't blame me?" Cheryl asked tentatively in a trembling voice. Her mother had always said as much, but Cheryl never believed her. But somehow, this time was different. Cheryl didn't know exactly why, but as she stared into her mother's eyes, she saw no blame—only love.

Charlotte's face broke out into one of the biggest smiles Cheryl had ever seen. Cheryl slowly returned the smile and then started to laugh. She wasn't sure exactly why she was laughing, but it sure felt good. Charlotte laughed in response, until they were both laughing so hard they couldn't catch their breath. Predictably, Charlotte began coughing and sputtering. Cheryl stopped laughing instantly, concerned for her mother. Although Charlotte was unable to speak at the moment, she indicated with her hands that she was okay, but just needed to calm down for a few minutes.

Cheryl watched Charlotte like a mother hen until she started to recover and regain some of her color.

"Are you okay now?"

Charlotte nodded and indicated to Cheryl to get her a glass of water. She still wasn't quite able to speak. On the way into the kitchen, Cheryl thought back to what her mother had said when she had first mentioned Joy's name. If her mother had had high sugar during her pregnancies, which then reverted to normal, then maybe, just maybe, Cheryl wasn't doomed. Perhaps she'd keep her appointment with Dr. Lang after all.

Charlotte settled herself down in front of the TV for the evening. Cheryl decided that she needed a good escape and went over to the bookshelf, where she kept her stash of romantic and mystery novels. She picked up a book by Nicholas Sparks called *Nights in Rodanthe*. As she read into the evening, she realized how little she knew about her mom's youth. *How did Mom and Dad meet?* she wondered, surprised that she'd never asked that of her mother before. It was really hard to picture her mother as a young woman. Even long before she became disabled, her earliest memories of her mother were of her coughing and constantly having to stop and catch her breath. It was hard to picture her running free on a beach or in a field. One of these days, she'd have to ask her about those things.

Cheryl drifted off to sleep. She dreamed about her father. He was alive. He had come to her wedding reception. Everyone was dancing, and he just walked in. He asked her to dance. She wanted him to meet her new husband. She searched all over the reception hall but couldn't find her husband. She became frantic and started searching the grounds, asking everyone if they had seen him. Then she turned around, and her father had vanished.

She tried to go back into the reception hall, but all the entrances were locked. She remembered a cellar door she could get into around the back. But when she went to the back of the building, it was a strange building that she had never seen before. She was totally lost. She was no longer in a wedding gown. She needed to call someone, but she couldn't find her cell phone or her purse. Had someone stolen her purse?

She looked for a familiar building or street. Perhaps she could find a pay phone. She thought she saw one up the street. She noticed that the phone was off the hook and making that horribly annoying sound. She kept hanging it up, but she couldn't get a dial tone—just that horrible noise, which droned on and on. She woke up, but she could still hear the phone. Her mother must've knocked the receiver off the phone in the next bedroom. She could hear the loud noise as if it were in her own room.

Cheryl staggered up and went into her mother's room to find her sleeping soundly. She picked up the receiver, replaced it, straightened out her mother's blankets, listened to her breathing for a few minutes, and then went back into her own bedroom.

How long had she been sleeping? And what in heaven's name had that dream been about? She had no clue. Cheryl looked at the clock. It was eleven thirty. She went into the bathroom to brush her teeth. In the mirror, she noticed that her eyes were red and puffy from crying earlier. She thought about the fact that she might be a little diabetic. She figured she could handle it. She had to, because she had to take care of her mother.

As she brushed her teeth, she remembered the peach Snapple she'd had earlier in the day. It really hadn't been half bad. Maybe she could do the diet drinks after all. Tomorrow she'd go to the supermarket, and get some diet Snapple, and some Splenda. She had an appointment with the doctor in four days. She was definitely going to keep it.

Chapter Five

May 2005

Cheryl sat in the exam room, nervously awaiting the doctor's arrival. A zillion questions were running through her mind. She didn't know where to start. Dr. Lang walked in the room, again wearing jeans and Docksiders. "How's it going, Cheryl?"

"I'm really nervous about my test results. You know, my dad had diabetes, and he died of a heart attack when he was in his early forties. I haven't slept very well since I got the lab results. Am I gonna die real early?"

"Slow down, Cheryl, and take a deep breath. First of all, you don't have diabetes—yet. Hold on. Hold on. Let me explain a few things first, and then you can ask some questions, okay?"

Cheryl nodded.

"At the present time, it appears that you have something called glucose intolerance, which—"

Cheryl interrupted, "Yeah, that's what my mother said."

"Glucose intolerance often leads to diabetes if we don't catch it early. So if you do nothing, you'll certainly become diabetic. Maybe not this year or next, but certainly by your forties."

"What can I do to prevent it?"

"Slow down, Cheryl. What do you think is the most common cause of adult onset diabetes?"

Cheryl shrugged.

"Obesity is the biggest reason that we have so many diabetics today," Dr. Lang continued. "What we have realized, though, is that many people can be spared the disease if we address it soon enough. Over the past few years, experts have lowered the ranges of normal for both glucose and cholesterol. Do you know why?"

Cheryl shrugged again.

Dr. Lang carried on. "Some people will tell you that it's so the pharmaceutical companies can sell more drugs."

"Yeah, I've heard that," answered Cheryl.

"Well, the truth of the matter is that it's so we can make earlier diagnoses and help prevent the secondary complications of these diseases. With the older, higher standards of acceptable glucose levels, some patients weren't deemed diabetic until they were already showing manifestations of the disease, like peripheral neuropathy."

"What's that?"

"The nerves of the feet get inflamed and painful for no apparent reason."

"That doesn't sound very pleasant."

"None of the complications of diabetes are pleasant. But the good news is that if you take your diagnosis seriously enough, you can help prevent those complications. In fact, I will go one step further and tell you that it's possible, if you take the right steps, for you to never develop diabetes."

"Is that really true?" Cheryl was getting truly excited. Maybe she wouldn't get diabetes after all.

"Yes, it can be true … but I have to tell you that it's more the exception than the rule."

"Why is that?"

"Well, let me ask you a question. How successful have you been in losing weight in the past?"

"Not very."

"So how many diabetics do you think are successful in not only losing a sufficient amount of weight, but in keeping it off?"

"Not many."

"We need to do another blood test today, called a hemoglobin A1C, that measures your glucose control over a three-month period. If that's normal, or near normal, then we can surely call you glucose intolerant, and not diabetic. But regardless, we need to begin treatment today if you want to try to avoid becoming outright diabetic."

"What do I have to do?"

"The most important thing you have to do is to take your health seriously enough to begin changing your eating habits. Have you stopped drinking your calories?"

"Almost," Cheryl replied a little sheepishly.

"Well, the good news is that you didn't gain any weight this month. That's the first place to start. Not gaining any weight is very important."

Cheryl breathed a sigh of relief. When she had gotten on the scale earlier and saw that she still weighed the same 235 pounds, she thought the doctor would be angry with her. But Dr. Lang wasn't.

"Let me ask you this: how much weight do you think you should lose in a month?"

"I don't know … maybe ten pounds?"

"Actually, ten pounds is too much," Dr. Lang replied. "I wouldn't want you to lose any more than three to four pounds in a month. For good health, you need to be more patient."

"Only three or four pounds?" Cheryl queried. "That doesn't seem like very much."

"Would you be happy if, a year from now, you had lost forty-eight pounds?"

Cheryl vigorously nodded her head in the affirmative.

"Well, think about it: four pounds per month for twelve months is forty-eight pounds."

"I guess you're right."

"What you have to realize is that all the ads you've seen on TV are basically lies. I'm sure you've seen ads that promise ten pounds of weight loss in just fourteen days, or something close to that. We already talked about there being approximately 3,600 calories in one pound, which means that there are 36,000 calories in ten pounds. So you would have to eat 36,000 calories less than your body required to lose ten pounds. Now, if we assume that you presently need 2,000 calories a day to maintain your present weight, and you stop eating completely by going on a fast, at the end of ten days, you will not have eaten 20,000 calories, and at the end of fourteen days, that would be 28,000 calories. That would still be 8,000 calories short of the 36,000 to achieve a ten-pound weight loss … and who's going to eat nothing at all for ten whole days?"

Dr. Lang was scribbling these numbers on the paper covering the exam table as she spoke so that Cheryl could follow what she was saying.

"So if we are realistic, and you cut back 500 to 600 calories per day, then you could actually expect to lose one pound in about six or seven days." Dr. Lang proceeded to do the calculations on the table paper: 600 x 6 = 3,600, or 500 x 7 = 3,500.

Cheryl agreed that from that perspective, the weight-loss claims did seem a bit unrealistic.

"But there's another reason that you don't want to lose weight too fast."

"What's that?" Cheryl was becoming a bit more curious.

"You slow down your metabolism."

"I don't understand. I mean, I'm familiar with the word "metabolism," but I thought that you're born with a set metabolism."

"Actually not. We are able to influence it. Let me explain. 'Metabolism' refers to the physical and chemical processes that your body requires to maintain itself.

Your heart beating, your brain thinking, your stomach digesting, and your muscles working are just a few of those activities. Each of these activities requires energy—calories. So when we talk about speeding up or slowing down your metabolism, we're really referring to the rate at which these processes burn calories.

"One of the many reasons that some longtime smokers are very thin is that their hearts and lungs are working so hard to do their jobs, they are burning hundreds of more extra calories per day."

Cheryl thought about her mother, and how thin she had been even before her appetite became so poor. Cheryl was starting to understand, but still wasn't fully on board. She nodded pensively as Dr. Lang continued.

"On the other hand, when the body doesn't get the energy it requires right then and there, and has to start breaking down fat and muscle cells to get it, it switches gears and uses a different pathway in order to conserve energy, and thereby burn fewer calories. So when you diet and drastically reduce your calorie consumption, your body actually becomes more efficient at holding onto the fat."

"I'm confused," Cheryl interjected. "You're telling me if I eat a whole lot less, my body holds onto the fat even more?"

"Not exactly." Dr. Lang paused, seeming to gauge how deeply she should delve into her explanation. After a few seconds, she continued. "I want to discuss a few other things with you today, so I'm going to ask you to pick up a chapter at the front desk that will hopefully clarify the role of metabolism so that we can move on now and cover a little bit more ground. For the moment, can you just accept the fact that dieting can slow your metabolism?"

Cheryl nodded tentatively.

"There's another reason that you don't want to go on a diet. I don't suppose you have any idea what that might be?"

Cheryl shook her head. "I haven't a clue."

"As I said to you on your first visit, when you go on a diet, you go off a diet." Dr. Lang looked at Cheryl to see if she remembered.

"Yes, I remember." She also thought about how unhappy she had been after that visit.

Dr. Lang continued, "So in essence, while you've been dieting, you've done nothing about changing any of your eating habits in the long run. It's important to understand that to lose weight and keep it off, you have to change habits. Diets providing rapid weight loss don't encourage that lifestyle adjustment. You're not doing anything long enough to establish any lasting behavioral modification.

"And, believe it or not, there's even another reason why you don't want to lose weight too fast."

Cheryl's interest was piqued. She couldn't believe there were so many disadvantages to losing weight quickly.

"If you lose weight too fast, your skin doesn't have a chance to shrink with you. Have you ever seen a person after they've had gastric bypass surgery?"

Cheryl shook her head.

"Well, all I can say is that it's often not pretty—loose skin hanging everywhere."

Cheryl had no difficulty imagining what that might look like, and she certainly didn't want to experience the reality of it … but losing weight that slowly was going to take forever, and Cheryl still wasn't sure she had the patience.

"Doctor Lang, I get your point, but if I only lose a few pounds a month, it's going to take me forever to lose all the weight I need to get rid of."

"You agreed earlier that losing forty-eight pounds in a year would make you happy. Right?"

Cheryl nodded.

"Do you think if you could actually see the weight coming off, that it would make it a little easier to be a bit more patient?"

"Absolutely!"

"Okay, so let me explain how that's going to work. But first, let me ask you a question. How many pounds do you think you can gain or lose in one day due to fluid retention?"

Cheryl thought of how bloated she felt when she got her period. "Two pounds?"

"Would you believe five pounds?"

"Really?"

"Yup, five pounds in one day. It depends on a lot of things. The obvious one is when you're premenstrual. But also, salt intake plays a big role. If you eat Chinese food for dinner, you might weigh a whole lot more the next morning than you did the previous one. Now, if you can lose or gain five pounds in one day, how easy is it to see a three- or four-pound weight loss in one month?"

Cheryl shrugged. She wasn't sure what was expected of her in response.

"It would be kind of difficult. Don't you agree?"

Cheryl agreed, but wasn't sure where the doctor was coming from.

"Most experts would have you weigh yourself once a week or once a month, but no more. I disagree. I think you should weigh yourself often, even as much as three or four times a day. What you want to determine is your dry and wet weight. Let me give you an example. Today, you weighed 235 pounds, but tomorrow morning, you might weigh only 232 pounds. Premenstrually, you might weigh 237 pounds. If you weigh yourself often, you'll find that the lowest number you ever see on the scale is your dry weight, and the highest number you see is your wet weight. When you begin to lose some real weight, you'll start to see a new low, and your higher number will drop as well. On the contrary, if you gain any real pounds, the reverse is true. Do you have a scale at home?"

"No, I threw them all away a number of years ago."

"I suggest that you go buy one. It will be really helpful. It's wonderful feedback whenever you see a new low. You might not see it again for a number of days, but then it'll start appearing more often. Frequent weigh-ins are the only way to get real feedback on your actual weight loss. If you come back a month from now not having weighed yourself during that entire time, and it happens to be closer to your period, you'll be mighty disappointed if it appears that you haven't lost any weight—when in fact, you may have truly lost three or four pounds."

"That would be really frustrating!" Cheryl knew what that felt like, so she was beginning to understand the benefits of Dr. Lang's advice. She knew for sure that she would personally benefit from that kind of feedback. Proof of her success would really help her be a bit more patient. She'd get a scale this weekend.

"So getting back to the task at hand, the first step in this process of changing habits is getting rid of the soda, juice, and sugar in your coffee. Do you think you can do that?"

"I do. I really think I can do that."

"Okay, so let's move to the second step. Did you know that most significantly overweight people eat only two meals a day?"

"Really? That's interesting ... 'cause I usually don't manage to eat breakfast most of the time."

"Have you ever noticed that it's the thin people who are always eating?"

"You know, I hadn't really given it much thought, but Tina and Janie, two of my co-workers, are always eating, and they're skinny as rails."

"I guess you figured they were just lucky and had fast metabolisms?"

Cheryl nodded again.

"Well, guess what? Eating all the time is what makes their metabolisms fast."

Cheryl started to open her mouth to say something, but Dr. Lang held up her hand to stop her.

"I know. I know. There's that word 'metabolism' again. Just try to accept for the moment that not eating frequently slows the metabolism, and eating all the time speeds it up. Okay?"

"Okay."

"Now, scientific studies have compared two groups of people that are similar in age, height, weight, and so on. Then they gave both groups exactly the same amount of calories—but one group ate two larger meals a day, and the other ate five smaller meals a day. The two-meal group stayed the same weight or gained weight, and the five-meal group lost weight. As a matter of fact, I just read an interesting statistic that, if you don't eat breakfast, you burn 300 fewer calories a day than someone who does. So, your second task is to eat breakfast."

"That's it? Don't drink my calories and eat breakfast. Nothing else?"

"Well, nothing else relating to diet. I do want to start you on a medication."

"But I thought I didn't have diabetes, so why do I have to take medication?"

"You don't want to get diabetes, right?"

Cheryl shook her head.

"This medication helps prevent you from getting diabetes. It's called Actos. It not only helps to prevent diabetes in some people, but it also helps to prevent the complications of the disease in those who already have it. I promise that if you can lose sufficient weight, and keep it off, you won't have to take this medication anymore."

Cheryl wasn't happy about taking pills—especially pills that wouldn't help her lose weight—but she really didn't want diabetes. She'd take the medication.

"And Cheryl, pick up the additional chapters of my book at the front desk, okay? They cover today's discussion."

Cheryl nodded.

"In fact, make it a habit to do so at the end of each visit. I find that an awful lot of patients get nervous when they're here in the office and forget most of what I tell them. Those chapters will help reinforce what you learn."

Cheryl did pick up the additional chapters and shoved them in her purse.

She left the doctor's office feeling a lot better than she had going in. Since it was an evening appointment, she went straight home afterward.

Cheryl came into the house with a smile on her face, and Charlotte breathed a visible sigh of relief.

"Mom, I don't have diabetes, and the doctor said that if I can lose some weight and take these pills"—she waved a prescription in the air—"I may never get it."

"So, did she have any diet suggestions?"

"Well, she told me I shouldn't drink my calories. That's why I got all those diet drinks last week. And, hey Mom—they're for me, not you. You need the calories."

Charlotte grinned wryly. "Anything else?"

"Well, she also told me that I needed to start eating breakfast."

"That's it?"

"Yup—she said that's all I have to do for now to begin creating new eating habits." Charlotte looked at her daughter quizzically.

"What a weird diet," she finally said. "Dr. Lang didn't say anything about your Snickers bars? You did tell her about the Snickers?"

Cheryl tried to avoid her mother's gaze.

"You didn't tell her, did you?"

Cheryl shook her head.

"Cheryl, how could you? You know you shouldn't be eating all that sugar."

Cheryl went into her room to change her clothes in an attempt to avoid her mother's query. Her mother followed in her wheelchair and just glared at her while she was changing.

"Okay, okay—I'll tell you what, Mom. You give up your cigarettes for good, and I'll give up my Snickers."

Cheryl could see her mother contemplating this request. "You've got a deal, daughter. What if you cheat?"

"What if you cheat?"

"Let's think about possible penalties for cheating. They've got to be consequential."

"I'll think about it, Mom."

"I will too." With that said, Charlotte headed back into the living room.

Just as Cheryl finished changing, the phone rang. It was Teresa.

"Sooo, how'd you make out at the doctor's today?"

"Actually, okay. I feel a lot better about things. My mom and I were just in the midst of making a deal. She'll give up her cigarettes if I give up my Snickers. We both agreed, but we haven't figured out what to do if either of us cheats. What do you think?"

"Hmmm, let me think about it."

"That was my response. I'm still thinking."

"How about this: if either one of you cheats, you get to call all the other's friends and report to them that they cheated. So all of your friends and your mom's friends have to know about the deal."

"I like that. I'll tell Mom."

They said their good-byes, and Cheryl put down the receiver. Her mother, who had been sitting right behind her, liked Teresa's idea too. They both agreed to share their deal with everyone. Cheryl made a mental note to try to get home a little early on Friday to make sure all Charlotte's bridge buddies knew about the deal, so they would stop bringing her cigarettes.

That settled, Cheryl went into the kitchen to throw something together for dinner. As she stared at the mostly empty fridge, she remembered her promise to eat breakfast in the morning. She closed the fridge and opened all the cupboards. The shelves were pretty bare. Eating breakfast was not going to be so easy!

She thought of the title of the chapter that Dr. Lang had given her—"Step 2 and Why It's So Important"—and hoped that it would help her figure out what to do next.

She found a package of macaroni and cheese and some leftover KFC lurking in the back of the refrigerator. That would do for now.

Over dinner, Cheryl told her mother about her plans to buy a scale and get her prescription filled. Charlotte was supportive of her daughter, but seemed especially tired and distracted.

When Charlotte went to bed early, Cheryl ran to the corner store to get some fruit yogurt and a granola bar for breakfast. She was proud of herself. She wasn't routinely reading labels yet, so she didn't take notice of all the sugar in her choices. That was okay, though; eating breakfast was the important new step.

Cheryl decided to curl up in bed early in order to read about Step 2. She wanted to do it right this time. Dr. Lang had said that many people fail through lack of knowledge. Cheryl might fail again, but it wasn't going to be because she didn't know enough!

What more did Cheryl learn?

STEP 2: EAT BREAKFAST
And Why It's So Important
By
Nikki Lang, MD

Eating breakfast, preferably before you leave the house for work, is the important second step in forming healthy eating habits.

Breakfast is an extremely important meal. Just as the name implies, it is when you break your fast. You're giving your body fuel for the day so that it doesn't remain in fasting mode.

If you already eat breakfast every day, great. For those of you who don't ordinarily eat breakfast, let's discuss your objections, and how we can overcome them.

Objection 1: I'm not hungry.
Objection 2: I don't have time.
Objection 3: There's no food in the house.
Objection 4: I hate breakfast food.

What's interesting is that Objection 1, not being hungry, is probably the easiest habit to change. Objections 2, 3, and 4 are a little more difficult. Once you start eating breakfast on a regular basis, even if it's just for a week or two, your body will quickly respond, and you will get hungry in the morning. In fact, you might even get hungry again a few hours later. This is your body letting you know that it's time to eat yet again.

The most difficult problem to overcome is probably going to be that there's no appropriate food in the house—Objection 3. That, of course, requires another habit change: making sure to stop at the store on a regular basis so that you always have something in the house to eat for breakfast.

Objection 4 is a little easier to overcome. Breakfast does not have to consist of Western-type "breakfast food." It's unimportant what the content of breakfast is. Many cultures eat the same types of food for breakfast as they do for lunch and dinner. The choice of content is yours. That leftover stir-fry will work just fine. You just have to eat something—which of course, still requires that there be some food in the house.

Objection 2, not having enough time, is primarily a rationalization. Let's examine this excuse. Ask yourself this question: How long does it really take to pour and eat a bowl of cereal, and then grab a piece of fruit on the way out the door? Five minutes? Maybe? With a minimum of effort, I think you can find five minutes to have breakfast. What, you don't like cereal? Then eat leftovers, as suggested under Objection 4. (Anything is better than nothing!) It really doesn't matter initially what's in your breakfast; the first step is to make sure you have it. As you become more accustomed to eating breakfast and then wanting breakfast, it will become a bit easier to plan a better breakfast.

So why is breakfast so important? Most obese people eat one or two larger meals per day. Somehow, they think they're doing themselves a favor by skipping meals. This is not true—in fact, they are doing themselves tremendous harm.

People who are thin tend to eat all the time. Their high metabolisms aren't entirely natural; smaller, more frequent meals actually speed up the metabolism. You've probably heard it before: eat small and often.

On the surface, such a statement may seem contrary to what you've always thought. "Eat often?" But isn't eating less better than eating more? Well, that's true, but we aren't discussing eating more calories. We're discussing distributing the same amount of calories across several smaller meals.

Scientific studies have shown that eating a certain number of calories per day in one or two meals burns fewer calories than eating the same amount of calories spread throughout the day in five or more meals.

Without getting terribly scientific, when the body doesn't receive any fuel for extended periods of time, it reverts to fasting mode. It figures out how best to conserve energy: what energy it can store, how to store that energy, and how to use as little energy as possible.

So if, during the day, you eat very little or nothing, your body will be very busy conserving. After you eat a great big evening meal, your body will only use what few calories it needs for the metabolism of a sleeping body, and store the rest as it again reverts to fasting mode several hours after dinner. Nor will it give up many of those extra calories the next day, because it's again busy conserving energy while you remain fasting.

On the other hand, if you give your body a small amount of fuel at a time, it becomes more wasteful. It doesn't hold on to its calories, because it expects more to arrive shortly. The body shifts into the normal way of obtaining calories, which ends up burning more. So, frequently, by the end of the day, you'll have burned more calories than you've eaten (if, of course, your meals are small).

For now, try to keep the calorie count of any new meal that you add within the recommended caloric limits: 350 calories for women and 450 calories for men, plus or minus 50 calories. If you don't have a calorie-counting book, I suggest you get one. It is important to educate yourself along the way. In a short period of time, you will have memorized the values of the foods you regularly come in contact with.

In Summary

STEP 1: **Stop drinking your calories.**

STEP 2: **Eat breakfast**

Chapter Six

May 2005

Breakfast never happened. Nor did the prescription get filled.

At about three in the morning, Cheryl was awakened by her mother's troubled breathing. Cheryl called 911. An ambulance came and took her mother to the hospital, with Cheryl following anxiously behind. She spent the wee hours of the morning pacing the floors of Methodist Hospital—first in the waiting room of the ER, and then in the intensive-care unit. It seemed that her mom had gone into heart failure again, and because of her chronic obstructive pulmonary disease or COPD in doctor jargon, she was having trouble breathing on her own.

At six in the morning, she finally got to see her mom, who was on a respirator. The physicians explained to Cheryl that her mother's lungs had again filled with fluid. They thought that maybe Charlotte had slacked off on taking her medication regularly—they weren't sure. It was always bad news when Charlotte had to be put on a ventilator, because it was so hard to get her off it again.

Cheryl didn't stand too close to her mother's bed. Charlotte seemed to be resting, and Cheryl didn't want to disturb her. She listened to the steady whooshing of the respirator. Her mom looked really white, except for that bluish tinge she always had from her lung disease. The doctors said she'd be all right, but Cheryl always got really nervous whenever her mother ended up in the hospital. *What if Mom doesn't come home again?*

Charlotte opened her eyes. She couldn't talk because of the endotracheal tube. But her eyes seemed to smile when she caught a glimpse of her daughter in the room.

Cheryl saw her mother's eyes open and moved to her bedside. She squeezed her mother's hand, and Charlotte squeezed back.

"Oh, Mom, what am I going to do with you?" Cheryl's eyes glistened. "The doctors told me you haven't been taking your medication the way you're supposed to, and that's why this happened. What am I supposed to do with you? Do I have to quit my job and watch over you 24–7?"

Charlotte squeezed her daughter's hand even tighter with what little strength she had. At the sight of her daughter's distress, her eyes began to moisten as well.

She tried to shake her head in an answer to her daughter's question, but it was difficult because of the respirator.

Cheryl responded, "I'm just not ready for you to leave me yet. Do you understand that you have to follow the doctor's instructions to a T? You promise?"

Charlotte's nod was barely perceptible, but it was there. Cheryl leaned over and kissed her mother's hand. "Please get better," she murmured.

The interchange had exhausted Charlotte, and her eyes fluttered closed. Cheryl stood by her mother's bedside for several more minutes until the fingers she clasped in her hand became slack. Charlotte had drifted into sleep.

Cheryl went back to the waiting room and called the office. It was still too early for anyone to be there, but she left a message on the voice mail that she wouldn't be in today. She picked up a magazine and began flipping pages. She wasn't really looking at anything; she just needed something to do with her hands.

She must have drifted off to sleep, because she was startled by a sudden keening sound in the room. A wretched-looking adolescent had collapsed into an older man's arms. The girl rocked back and forth while her father held her, trying unsuccessfully to console her. He too had tears pouring down his face. He looked away, toward the other wall, as though he didn't want Cheryl to see his tears. A nurse came in and asked the man if he wanted to spend a few minutes with his wife before they moved her body from the room. He nodded in the affirmative. He hugged his daughter even tighter and began talking quietly and soothingly in her ear. They walked out of the waiting room together, leaning on each other for support.

Cheryl couldn't help thinking that it could've been her mother who had died. She jumped up and rushed back to her mother's bedside, then sagged in relief. Charlotte was fine. The respirator whooshed as Cheryl watched her mother's chest rise in response. She thought about what her mother's life had been like for the past ten to fifteen years: multiple visits to doctors, numerous hospitalizations, oxygen tanks, and wheelchairs. Most of Charlotte's life was now spent within the confines of their home; any outing beyond the living room was a major production. Cheryl's mother had her good friends, who were more than willing to come to their house. They were funny and warm people who really looked after her. Cheryl didn't want that for herself, though. She wanted more ... but would she ever get more?

She was admittedly envious of Wendy, Susan, and Carol, who had husbands. Well, Wendy wasn't married yet, but she would be soon, and her fiancé was really great. He was a bit on the serious side, so he didn't always get their jokes, but he was so caring and good to Wendy. He worked in a bank and was always getting promotions. He'd probably be very successful one day. Wendy really deserved it.

And what about Susan? She was about to have her second child. Cheryl was excited for her friend, but part of her wondered if she would always have to just be "Aunt Cheryl."

Yes, she was jealous. She wanted a family too. But that really wasn't going to happen if she never went out and never met anyone new. Oh, occasionally she'd go out with the girls, but who wanted to meet someone in a bar? Besides, who would ever want a fat girl? Even fat guys weren't particularly interested in fat women. If she were completely honest with herself, she would have to admit that she really wasn't very attracted to fat men either.

She was beginning to understand her outburst in the dressing room a couple of months ago. She really did want to change, but she was afraid she wouldn't be able to do it. It was really depressing to consider that the rest of her life might not be a whole lot different than her mom's. What a sobering thought. What if she did get diabetes and lost a foot—or her kidneys? What would life be like on dialysis? *No—that isn't going to happen to me! I can't let that happen to me!* Cheryl made up her mind that somehow, some way, she was going to change.

Cheryl spent the rest of the day in the hospital. She didn't want to leave until she was absolutely certain that her mother was okay. By the time she walked out the hospital doors, she was absolutely starving, as well as exhausted. She went to a nearby McDonalds to grab some dinner. She realized that she hadn't eaten all day except for several black coffees—yeah, yeah, with sugar in them. She shook her head when she remembered her broken promise to eat breakfast. She got a double cheeseburger, large fries, and a large Diet Sprite. (They didn't have ginger ale.) By the time she'd gotten home, the fries were gone.

The phone was ringing as she walked in the door. It was Teresa. She wanted to know why Cheryl hadn't been at work. Cheryl brought her friend up to date on her mother's health and declined a trip to the shore.

"I understand," Teresa said, and the warmth in her voice made Cheryl feel even more like crying. "Is there anything I can do?"

Cheryl turned down any help or company, saying she was exhausted and would probably be in bed by eight thirty.

As fatigued as Cheryl was, she had difficulty falling asleep. She couldn't help worrying about her mother and all the things she needed to do and hadn't managed to get done. She still hadn't gotten her prescription filled. She hadn't done any grocery shopping. And where was she going to get a bathroom scale? She had to go into work tomorrow, so she'd have to stop off at the hospital before and after work to check on her mom. She'd drive rather than take the bus, which meant she'd have to pay for parking all day. Although not horribly expensive, it went against her natural instincts of economy. Maybe she could go shopping after work and go to the hospital after, now that she didn't have to rush home to look after her mother.

Cheryl still hadn't gotten Wendy's wedding present, and the wedding was next weekend. She hadn't even scheduled an appointment to get her hair done for the big day, much less bought a dress—even though she was a bridesmaid. Fortunately, Wendy had insisted that they wear whatever they wanted. She didn't want all her friends to have to spend money on a particular color dress that they might never wear again. Cheryl knew that whatever each of them wore, no matter how disparate, Wendy would somehow make it work. She was amazing like that.

Cheryl was so lucky to have such great friends. So why was she crying again? She turned over in bed and punched the mattress. She wanted to stand at the end of that aisle as a bride, not as just another bridesmaid.

"Oh, Mom," she cried out. "Please be okay. I need you. You have to help me get through this. I really want to lose the weight this time. I really do. But I need your help. Please, Mama. Get better! Please." Cheryl sobbed her heart out. When she had no tears left, she dropped into an exhausted sleep.

The following day, Cheryl learned that her pleas had been answered. Arriving at the hospital before work, she found her mother had already been weaned off the respirator. Thank God. Charlotte still wouldn't be going home for a few days, but the good news gave Cheryl the renewed energy she'd needed to get all her tasks completed.

Chapter Seven

June 2005

Cheryl had been right: the wedding was beautiful. Wendy had the florist make multicolored bouquets with different predominant colors. Wendy and the florist agreed that in order to tie everything together, they would attach large ribbon lengths of varying colors to each of the bouquets, blending the flowers with the dresses. The florist matched each bridesmaid with a bouquet, then chose ribbons accordingly. Wendy then suggested a particular order for the procession. It worked.

Cheryl cried; she wasn't quite sure whether she felt happier for her friend or sorrier for herself. She enjoyed herself, dancing a lot—especially when a partner wasn't required. She actually got a little tipsy. Normally, she just didn't like the taste of alcohol, but she ended up drinking several glasses of champagne.

Cheryl's mom was back home from the hospital, with the help of a visiting nurse who came three days a week. Charlotte was too weak to resume her card games, so Cheryl wasn't yet sure if all her friends knew the "no cigarettes, no Snickers" deal she had struck with her mother. She wasn't too worried, though. She didn't think they'd get her any cigarettes so soon after being in the hospital.

Cheryl had finally gotten her prescription filled and was taking it faithfully every morning. She was always so bad at remembering to take pills, so she made a promise to herself that she couldn't brush her teeth in the morning until she took her pill. Now, every time she reached for her toothbrush, she would think *pill*, and if she hadn't yet taken it, she made herself put down the toothbrush, take her pill, and then resume brushing her teeth. It was working; she hadn't forgotten in over a week.

She had also purchased a scale—a digital one with big numbers that couldn't be denied. The doctor was right: her weight did fluctuate, between 232 and 237. Cheryl was very pleased with herself. Yesterday morning, when she'd gotten on the scale, it had read 231—her first new low.

Although Cheryl knew her mother really wasn't in a position to break their bargain, Cheryl was keeping her side. She had decided that while her mother was in the hospital, she would have a small, private ceremony to truly commit to giving up her Snickers bars. She'd gone into her bedroom closet and pulled out the entire carton of Snickers that she kept for "emergencies." She then rooted around in the backyard shed and found a trowel. After a brief funeral, she left her Snickers to their eternal rest near the flowerbed—or at least she hoped it would be eternal. The ceremony had included a prayer that she'd have the strength to leave them there.

Breakfast was still something of a problem, but she was working on it. Somehow, mornings kept getting away from her, and she kept running out of time. She had started buying fruit and fruit yogurts to keep in the house, so she could grab something on the way out the door when she hadn't managed to eat by then. At least she could eat those on the bus. But sometimes, she didn't have anything in the house to grab. By the time she got to work, a busy day was usually under way—no time to eat. Still, she was getting better at it.

Oddly, Cheryl often found herself hungry again just a few hours after breakfast—like by ten thirty. So by lunchtime, she was starving. She felt as if she could eat an elephant. That didn't make any sense to her. In fact, sometimes she would grab a bag of chips if they were handy in the middle of the morning. She was certain Dr. Lang hadn't intended this.

But overall, she was pleased with herself. She was drinking diet drinks regularly, and was well stocked with Splenda. She had plenty at work, in her purse, and at home. It tasted fine to her. When out, she often just ordered plain iced tea and sweetened it with Splenda.

Cheryl was actually looking forward to her next doctor's appointment in a couple of weeks, eager to see how she was progressing. Dr. Lang had requested that she get her blood drawn a few days early so that the results would be available at the next office visit. Cheryl needed to have her sugar and insulin levels checked first thing in the morning before she ate. She was hoping her sugar would be normal. She wasn't quite sure why an insulin level was needed.

The next two weeks passed quickly. Cheryl's mom was back to her weekly bridge games, and Cheryl made sure that all of Charlotte's friends knew about the deal.

Cheryl also made progress in the food-shopping department. She asked Dr. Weiner if she could come to work a little early on Wednesdays, then leave a little earlier so she'd have time to get to the supermarket before dinnertime. If she got home too late, her mom wouldn't really eat anything.

Cheryl started spending just a little more time shopping, making sure the cabinets always had something to offer—especially for breakfast. She'd bought some of those Lean Cuisine dinners too, so she didn't have to always stop for dinner on the way home. She was beginning to realize what Dr. Lang had meant about so many other habits having to change.

Cheryl also found herself spending more time with her mother, since her mom had just recently come home from the hospital. This was just as well. Teresa had met a new guy a couple of weeks ago, and she didn't have a whole lot of free time to spend with Cheryl. Cheryl didn't know very much about him yet, but she figured if he stayed around long enough, she'd soon find out. Cheryl wanted all her friends to be happy, so she hoped that Teresa's new boyfriend worked out for her. But her hopes for her friend were tainted with depression. *Suppose Teresa gets married too? I'll be the only one who's still single … and it'll be obvious enough why.*

She sat up straighter and squared her shoulders. *I will not feel sorry for myself,* she thought.

She'd seen two more new lows on her scale. Her latest low was 229. She was making progress. In fact, she was losing weight—granted, not a whole bunch of weight, but she was losing and not depriving herself. Amazingly, she wasn't even on a diet. Her switch to diet drinks had begun just over a month ago, and it really hadn't been that difficult. She had reread Dr. Lang's article on acquired taste, so she was still staying away from all Pepsi, both regular and diet. She didn't want to mess with what was working. She realized that she had made a number of changes, but her life didn't feel particularly disrupted.

True, it had taken her over three weeks to get in the habit of having breakfast every day. But she was beginning to understand what the doctor had said about how many habits had to really change. For example, she couldn't eat breakfast every day if she didn't shop regularly as well. She just hoped she could keep up the routine.

Cheryl went in early Friday morning to Dr. Lang's office to get her blood drawn. She brought her large fruit yogurt and banana with her, which she ate after the test, while she walked the few blocks to work. She had gotten in and out of Dr. Lang's office so quickly, she was actually early for work. The entire office staff ribbed her about getting in early, asking what the occasion was. She told them about having her blood drawn and about her upcoming appointment.

"So," Tina asked, "how's the diet coming? No one's wanted to say anything in case you were upset about it, but I have to admit that we've all been wondering. One minute, you're drinking a diet soda, but the next minute, you're eating chips. You're certainly making us curious about this diet!"

"I'm not on a diet," Cheryl retorted. "I'm just working on changing a few habits. It's like that friend of yours said—you know, the waiter who plays ice hockey. It's more about attitude. I've just made a couple of small changes, and I'm actually losing weight!"

"You think you might really do it this time?"

"I'm not counting my chickens yet, but I'm at least feeling a little positive. The doctor told me that I'm not diabetic, I'm only glucose intolerant. If I change enough habits over time, I might be able to prevent myself from ever becoming diabetic. So I'm trying to just take it one step at a time."

"That's awesome," Tina said. "If there's anything I can do to help, please let me know, okay?"

"Sure," responded Cheryl, thinking to herself that no one could do this for her. But in the coming weeks, she would realize that a little help might be just what she needed.

Cheryl has begun to realize how many other habits need to change. Let's review some of them.

OTHER HABITS THAT NEED CHANGING
By
Nikki Lang, MD

Earlier, we discussed that changing eating habits requires hundreds of changes. What we eat is influenced by many behaviors. What you buy at the grocery store will dictate what you eat for breakfast, along with how long you've had it (is it still fresh?) and how it was stored.

In this very busy world of ours, it's hard to find enough time to go to the grocery store. Even when we get there, we usually rush up and down the aisles, grabbing only things that are familiar to us, rather than the right foods.

So what do you need to do? At least once a month, you need to spend that little bit of extra time in the supermarket. Begin looking for new possibilities. Read the package labels and figure out what might appeal to you. Explore the vegetable aisle. Look for some new and interesting vegetables. You don't need to purchase one the first time you see it, but make a note of the name and then research it over the next couple of weeks. What is it? How can it be prepared? Most of us, even if we don't have a computer at home, have access to one at work. Do an Internet search.

I remember the first time I saw a spaghetti squash. I had no clue what it was or what to do with it. I went home and researched it; I didn't actually purchase one until a month or so later. Subsequently, though, I've enjoyed it on a regular basis. Had I never taken the time to examine it in the supermarket and research it at home, I'd never have included it in my expanding diet repertoire.

Periodic extra time at the supermarket is a must.

As you explore these new foods, also give some thought to the packaging, amounts, and the way these foods need to be used and stored. Are you shopping for one, two, three, or more? Make sure your purchases—for example, frozen foods—can be separated into appropriate portions? Often, when we cook too much, we end up eating too much. Of course, as long as you plan for leftovers for other meals, this may not be a problem. Buying frozen vegetables in bags gives you a great deal more flexibility, because you can cook as small or as large a portion as you need without wasting the rest.

By planning ahead and separating food into appropriate portions before freezing it, you can also save a great deal of money by taking advantage of sales. If a family pack of meat or chicken is on sale, you should buy it, no matter how many are in your family—as long as you immediately package it into appropriate portions.

If you are shopping for one, it might be necessary to cut meats or other food items into even smaller pieces and package them individually. For example, depending on the size, you may want to cut chicken breasts in half, reducing their thickness by half (butterfly method), or possibly even in quarters. This way, if you forget to set frozen food out to thaw in the morning, you can quickly defrost it in the microwave when you get home.

You may want to invest in a small home vacuum packer. Food does truly remain far fresher for much longer when it is vacuum-packed.

How food is packaged and stored at home plays an important role in changing your eating habits for the better.

Another way to promote changes in your eating habits is spending some extra time on days off preparing foods for the rest of the week. Then, when you are much busier, you can grab stuff that's already prepared. This behavior requires a lot more discipline and planning, and I suspect that most people will not be so prepared. However, let me give you a little food for thought.

One day, you open your vegetable drawer in the fridge, and you notice a lot of stuff is starting to go bad. Stop before you throw all that stuff away. Much of it might be salvageable for vegetable soup. Instead of just tossing all that food, cut away the bad parts and cut the remainder into small pieces. Along with some onions and seasonings, throw it all into a large pot of water. Toss in a few bouillon cubes and let it simmer all day on the stove. Maybe add a few small pieces of other leftovers floating around in the fridge. After it's been cooking for several hours, give it a taste. If it's not flavorful enough, add some more seasonings or more bouillon. When the soup is finished, pour it into meal-size containers and put them in the freezer. Each of these containers now holds the basis for a quick meal. You can make each meal taste differently by adding other ingredients at the time of final preparation. Some of your experiments may end up being disasters, but you might actually discover some neat meals. Don't be afraid, even if you're not much of a cook. It's truly worth the effort. You were going to throw out those vegetables anyway.

Sometimes, when preparing a dinner, you may want to make a large roast or chicken or turkey breast. That way, when dinner is over, you can slice and separate the leftovers into appropriate portions, package them, and freeze them for later.

One of the reasons that the dieting program Jenny Craig has been so successful for many people over the short run is that they provide portion- and calorie-controlled meals. These meals are rather expensive, however, and they do nothing to help you to create your own habits. It is also unlikely that you will pay for Jenny Craig meals for the rest of your life.

A Lean Cuisine entrée, or some other prepackaged meal that fits into your caloric requirement, is certainly a reasonable alternative from time to time. Keeping some of these in your freezer for "emergencies" will help to keep you on track, but they are not a permanent answer for the long run. As you establish your new habits, the use of these prepared meals should become less frequent.

Changing your eating habits takes time, because it requires so many other habits to change as well. The trick, again, is not to change too many things at once. Change a few, and stick with those changes so that they are more likely to stick with you.

Undoubtedly, you'll have trouble establishing these new behaviors. It's okay—just keep plugging away. Little by little, you will make progress.

Chapter Eight

June 2005

Cheryl kept checking her watch all day. She couldn't believe she was looking forward to her doctor visit. The anticipation surrounding her previous visits had been quite different. Now, she was actually wondering what new changes were in store for her. She was eager to get on the scale and show the doctor that she had lost weight. *Imagine that—looking forward to getting on a scale!* Her appointment was for six in the evening, just in case any last-minute issues popped up at the end of the workday.

She was early for her appointment, but amazingly, the doctor was also running ahead of schedule. The small black assistant took Cheryl back to the scale to get weighed, and by this time, Cheryl had learned her name: Latisha. Even though Cheryl didn't know Latisha well, she felt like hugging the woman when she saw the results on the scale, which showed she had lost four pounds. She now weighed 231—progress! It wasn't the low she was getting at home, but she always weighed more in the evening.

Dr. Lang walked in the room with the chart. Her smile was almost as big as Cheryl's own. "Congratulations, Cheryl. You've lost four pounds. I'm very proud of you." Cheryl was very proud of herself.

"I have more good news," Dr. Lang continued. "You're not diabetic for sure, only glucose intolerant. The hemoglobin A1C that we did was just a smidgen over normal at 6.0. Your insulin levels are high, as expected. But your repeat fasting blood sugar was normal at 92."

Cheryl beamed. "Does that mean I can stop taking the medication?"

"No, it doesn't. When you lose sufficient weight, you can stop the medication."

Cheryl's smile drooped at the edges. "What's sufficient?"

"We'll know when your fasting insulin levels are normal. You see, many of the horrible side effects of diabetes come from the high insulin levels, not just the high sugars. Insulin resistance is another name for glucose intolerance. As you become more and more insulin resistant, which seems to correlate with weight gain, your insulin levels rise, and you are at greater risk for damage to the tissues.

So you really want to keep taking the medication to help protect your organs and blood vessels."

"I guess so," Cheryl answered, not really fully comprehending the explanation.

"So, how have you been doing with the changes that we've made so far?"

"Actually, pretty good. For the past week or so, I've eaten breakfast every morning, and I haven't had one regular soda or fruit drink for an entire month. Oh, and no sugar in my coffee."

"Has it been difficult?"

"Well, breakfast was hard. Half the time, I didn't have anything in the house to eat, but now, I have a weekly shopping routine that seems to be working. The only thing that bothers me is that by the middle of the morning, I get so hungry that I can't wait for lunch, so I end up eating a bag of potato chips or something. And I know that's not what I should be doing."

"Well, no, that's not ideal, but it's the perfect segue for our next topic. Do you remember when I talked about the study that had been done with two groups of people—one eating two meals a day, and the other five?"

Cheryl nodded.

"The reason you get hungry in the middle of the morning is that your body is telling you it wants food again. When you break your fast, you change your body's metabolism from a fasting state, and it now expects to be fed every three hours. So you should eat again at ten thirty."

Cheryl knew the doctor could tell she was crestfallen. She worked for a dentist. She did procedures all morning. How was she going to eat a meal?

Dr. Lang addressed Cheryl gently, clearly noticing her chagrin. "Let me ask you a question, Cheryl. How long does it really take to eat a sandwich, if you're not talking and have no interruptions?"

Cheryl thought about it for a few seconds. "Probably no more than five minutes."

"Exactly. We're all busy at work, but when it comes right down to it, most of us can find five minutes to eat a sandwich. I'd be willing to bet it takes longer to eat a bag of potato chips."

Cheryl laughed; Dr. Lang was probably right. "But you don't have to prepare a bag of potato chips," Cheryl retorted.

Dr. Lang smiled. "That's absolutely true. So the question is, how can you make sure that 'real food' is available when you want it?"

"I don't know. I get so tied up in the morning at work. I might realize I'm hungry, but I can't order anything because I'm in the middle of a procedure. And then, even if I do, someone has to go pick it up, or it has to be delivered. By the time my snack would arrive at the office, it would almost be lunchtime."

"How about keeping several takeout menus in the office with preplanned orders circled? That way, when you get tied up, you could maybe ask someone else to order your food for you at the appropriate time. In fact, when you arrive each day at the office, if you don't have your meal with you, why not make delivery arrangements before you even start your procedures? Then, if your lunch is delivered by ten thirty, you could eat half of it then and the other half at lunchtime."

Cheryl nodded slowly. This was starting to seem feasible.

"The simplest solution," Dr. Lang continued, "would be to bring your meals to work, but I realize that not all of us are that organized, so let me make other suggestions."

Cheryl nodded in agreement. "I have enough trouble getting breakfast; I'm not sure I could get it together enough to bring in my meals every day."

"I understand. But let me ask you this: Do you have a refrigerator at work?"

"We do."

"When you go grocery shopping, do you think you could buy some snacks to keep in the fridge for emergencies? That way, if things don't work out earlier in the day, you would have something to fall back on."

"Like what?"

"Sandwich fixings, soup, and salad stuff."

Cheryl considered the suggestion. "Hmmm ... I suppose I could do something like that." She also thought of the Lean Cuisine entrées that she kept in the freezer at home. Why not do something similar at work?

"Now, before we finish up, there is one more thing I would like to discuss. Would you agree that we human beings are such creatures of habit that we usually eat the same things all the time?"

"Oh, sure."

"So don't cringe too much when I tell you that I'd like you to start counting calories. It's not really as hard as it sounds. Since we do really often eat the same things, it becomes easier and easier to sort out the calories in any given meal. Whenever you add any new meals, I'd like you to try to keep them in the 300- to 350-calorie range. After a while, you'll get to know what ingredients add up to a 350-calorie sandwich, for example.

"Remember when we talked about knowledge being a very important part of doing a job well? Well, a large part of that information is knowing how much energy—specifically, the calorie count—is in the foods you eat. The more you know, the better your decisions will be. I'm not asking you to look up and count everything you eat all day at this point. Just make sure that when you add a new small meal to your diet repertoire, you're not adding one that has too many calories."

"How will I know how many calories are in something if it doesn't come in a package?"

"You need to get a calorie-counting book. You can get one at a library or any bookstore. I have one here in the office for convenience. It's seven dollars, and it's one of the better ones I've seen. It even lists all the fast foods."

"Is that it? Just figure out how to eat a 350-calorie meal at ten thirty in the morning?"

"And continue to eat breakfast every day, and make certain that you're not drinking your calories," Dr. Lang reminded Cheryl.

"Anything else?"

"Not today, but I'd like you to make another appointment in a couple of weeks. There are a couple of other things I want to discuss with you, but I don't want to burden you with too much information all at once."

Cheryl stopped at the front desk for the calorie-counting book on her way out. She glanced through it on the way home. The contents seemed pretty simple, and the book was small enough to fit in her purse.

By the time Cheryl had gotten home, it was pretty late, so she popped a couple of Lean Cuisines in the oven. As her food cooked, she flipped over the box and read the nutrition information: 270 calories each. *Not bad.* The one problem, though, was that she usually ended up eating most of her mother's as well.

Charlotte was watching *Wheel of Fortune*. Sometimes, she and Cheryl would compete to see who could solve the puzzle first. Her mom frequently beat Cheryl, as she did tonight.

Cheryl waited for *Wheel of Fortune* to be over before pushing her mother's chair toward the dinner table. "I'm not really that hungry," Charlotte said.

"Look, Mom. The doctor said I should be eating 300 to 350 calories per meal. These meals are 270 calories each. If you don't eat it, I will, and I'm not supposed to eat that much."

Cheryl sure knew how to push her mother's buttons. Charlotte ate a few small bites and washed it down with some water. "So what else did the doctor say?"

"My sugar was normal on Friday, but I still have to take the medication until I lose enough weight to bring down my insulin levels."

"I thought that diabetes made insulin levels too low, not too high."

"That's what I'd thought too. But she said something about glucose intolerance being the same as insulin resistance, and when that happens, your insulin levels are too high. I guess I'll have to ask Dr. Lang to explain it to me again. It's a bit confusing. I've got another appointment in a couple of weeks—I'll ask her about it then."

"So, what else did she tell you? Did you ever tell her about the Snickers bars?"

"No, Ma, I didn't tell her about the Snickers, and I don't plan to tell her about the Snickers. They're dead and buried." Quietly, so her mother wouldn't hear her, she murmured, "I hope."

"Did the doctor say anything else about what you're eating?" Charlotte managed to get another few bites of food in her mouth.

"Actually, yes. She told me that since I'm eating breakfast, I have to eat again at ten thirty in the morning."

"I'll be damned. This is, without a doubt, the strangest diet I've ever heard of. She keeps telling you to eat more? Cheryl, are you losing any weight?"

"Yep. I've lost four pounds since I saw her last month."

"I'll be damned," her mother muttered again. "Cheryl, honey, I'm sorry, but I really can't eat another mouthful."

"You did really well, Ma. You ate about half of it." Cheryl was really happy her mother couldn't finish it; she was still hungry. She didn't know how she'd ever be satisfied with a 350-calorie dinner.

Begin thinking about how you too can eat smaller, more frequent meals.

STEP 3, STEP 4: FITTING IN FIVE SMALL MEALS A DAY
By
Nikki Lang, MD

I cannot emphasize enough what an important role smaller, more frequent meals represent in a healthy lifestyle. These meals not only increase your metabolism, but they also decrease snacking and overeating.

Since Step 2 in this process is to eat breakfast, then it logically follows that Step 3 is to eat a small meal between breakfast and lunch. The easiest way to accomplish this is to divide lunch into two parts so that by the time you have eaten all of your lunch, you've already had three meals. If you normally eat a sandwich for lunch, eat half of it around ten thirty and eat the other half at lunchtime.

Since we generally eat our meals throughout an approximately twelve-hour period (breakfast around 7:00 AM and then dinner by 6:00 or 7:00 PM), then all our meals should be about three hours apart. So, if you had breakfast at 7:30 in the morning, then you should eat the first half of your sandwich around 10:30, and the second half at 1:30.

I can already hear your objections: "I usually eat lunch out." "I don't have time to eat in the morning." "There's no food near where I work." "I don't have time to make my own lunch." "My boss won't let me eat on the job." The potential hurdles go on and on. Each of these objections has a solution, so let me make a few suggestions.

The least expensive and most practical solution is to bring your own lunch (which could be dinner leftovers) and pack it for easy dividing. I realize this takes time and preparation, but it could be done the night before, rather than during an already rushed morning routine.

But since most of us are not that organized, let me make a few other suggestions. If you generally order out for lunch or go to a local restaurant or deli, order lunch at 10:00 (they won't be very busy) and have it delivered by

10:30. That way, you can eat half of it then, and the other half at lunchtime.

If you find that you're often so busy in the morning that stopping to look at a menu, picking something out, and making the call will take up too much time, then try a little preplanning. One lunchtime, or on some evening after work when you have a little extra time, stop in at all the local restaurants and pick up menus. Sit down with those menus and study them. Circle the items that you would prefer in combinations that will work for you. Look up the calories and mix and match your selections until you've come up with several workable combinations. Keep these menus in your desk at work. Then, when you're busy, all you have to do is to pull one out and make the call, or ask someone else to make the call. This will only take a couple of minutes. Remember, you're looking for a 700-calorie (for women) or 900-calorie meal (for men), because you're going to divide it in half.

Another possibility is making a little extra dinner on purpose the night before, then putting it aside for the next day. Even when you go out to dinner, you can order with the next day in mind—that's why the doggie bag was invented!

Patients tell me that they don't have time to eat in the middle of the morning, but in reality, preparation is the issue. If you already have your food, how long does it actually take to chew and swallow? Five minutes? Seven minutes?

One patient stated that he was frequently in confer-ences at the designated time. He agreed, however, that these meetings weren't so formal to preclude eating while working. He just wasn't in a position to order food in the middle of the conference. He realized that he could bring the food into the conference with him. I cannot speak to all the different circumstances surrounding your particu-lar job or employment. You should consider some of these suggestions and figure out what will work for you.

One problem-solving strategy is to pretend that your problem belongs to someone else. How would you help him or her solve it? We're usually much better at solving someone else's problems than our own. Most people are far smarter than they give themselves credit for; they just give up too easily. Rather than saying immediately that something is impossible, list your objections and then try to figure out how to get around them. Once you find the solution, all you have to do is implement it.

So far, I haven't advised you on the content of any meal, and I won't for some time. You do not as yet have sufficient information to always make a satisfying small meal within caloric limits. For now, just use the calorie count as a guide when creating new meals. There is no reason why cereal and fruit couldn't be the second meal of the day. It's quick and easy, and many offices have a kitchen, or mini-kitchen, where milk and cereal could be kept on hand. For that matter, store-bought prepared meals can work. Some patients tell me they keep sandwich fixings, soup, and salad ingredients in the office kitchen to make frequent meals easier.

We've now discussed four meals: breakfast, midmorning, lunch, and dinner. So where's the fifth? Well, dinner is actually the fifth meal of the day; we just haven't discussed the fourth yet.

A few hours before dinner, you should eat an appetizer. You want to eat your fourth small meal of the day at 4:30 or 5:00, then have your dinner by 7:30 or 8:00. I know you've been told it's not healthy to eat later in the evening. Well, remember, you're not eating a great big meal. You're only eating a small meal, and that small meal will provide just enough calories for you to burn while you sleep. Your heart still needs to beat; you still need to breathe. You are burning calories … just not that many. A small meal later in the evening is actually a perfect guard against evening snacking.

Okay, so how do we squeeze in that fourth meal? One easy way is to include it when you're making or ordering lunch. Triple the calories (to 1,050–1,350), and then divide the meal by three—a hoagie cut in thirds might even work! Or you could have breakfast in two parts, and then have lunch in two parts, with the second part at 4:30 or 5:00. Stop and pick something up on the way home. Grab a hearty salad, or soup, or half a sandwich, as soon as you walk in the door, but before you start preparing dinner. Many solutions exist; use the ones that are right for you.

Before changing subjects, I want to discuss the other benefits of eating more frequent, smaller meals; it's not just about metabolism. This meal plan actually helps to not only address other bad habits (like snacking on things you shouldn't between meals), but in many ways, it also helps you to eat less and eat healthier.

When we allow ourselves to get really hungry, we tend to overeat. When we're feeling starved, it doesn't take us very long to consume a large amount of food, and, unfortunately, the message that we've had enough to eat takes far longer. I'm sure you recall being admonished to eat more slowly, but quite frankly, no matter how slowly you eat or chew, it won't be slow enough for your body to catch up unless you pause between courses.

For example, we've all had the experience of going to a restaurant quite hungry, then ordering both an appetizer and a main course. After eating the appetizer, we are forced to wait, sometimes as much as thirty minutes, before dinner is served. And what happens? Although you were still starving after finishing the restaurant appetizer, you now find that you're no longer hungry, and that you've ordered far too much food. Had you been at home, you would have already plowed through the main course before this realization hit. The fourth meal of the day (your appetizer equivalent) will prevent that starving state and subsequent overeating. You will then discover that the small dinner you planned is more than adequate.

You may find that you start to get hungry a couple of hours before lunch, but it's not time for lunch, so you grab a bag of chips, pretzels, or some other snack food. These options really don't stave off your hunger that much, and you're still starving by the time lunch rolls around. In spite of the extra calories in the snack you consumed earlier, you'll be likely to overeat.

If you eat a small midmorning meal, you won't be terribly hungry for lunch, and a small lunch will suffice.

By eating every three hours or so, you never allow your-self to get to the "I feel like I could eat an elephant" state. The tendency to overeat diminishes. Interestingly, you'll find that your stomach will tell you when the three hours are up; you'll feel those first few twinges of hun-ger. You might also find it surprising that if you eat fewer than 300-350 calories, your hunger will come before the three hours are up, and if you're unable to eat by then, you'll be starving in another hour. So it's just as important to eat enough calories with each meal as it is to avoid eating too many.

Evening snacking in front of the TV is also likely to disappear under this plan. If you tend to nibble your way through the evening, you may want to plan your last two meals a bit later. If you've just eaten dinner at 8:30 or 9:00, snacking becomes much less of an issue.

One aspect of frequent meals is that if you're eating something really, really good, you can look forward to eating more of it at your next meal a few hours hence.

I recently had a patient return after almost a year on the five-meal plan who had lost a fair amount of weight (approximately 21 pounds). She stated that the plan really worked well for her, because if she really had to have that piece of chocolate cake, she could have it for one of her meals and still stick to her plan.

Let's review our steps:

> **Step 1:** **Stop drinking your calories.**
> **Step 2:** **Eat breakfast.**
> **Step 3:** **Eat a small meal between breakfast and lunch.**
> **Step 4:** **Eat an appetizer a few hours before dinner.**

It really doesn't matter whether you work on Step 4 before Step 3, but it is important to work on Steps 1 and 2 before proceeding with the others. It's too difficult to make progress on all four steps at the same time. Try leaping to the top of a ladder. Now try it one rung at a time. Which method is easier?

This is a process that has to be taken one step at a time. As we stated before, the more often you repeat a behavior, the sooner it will become a habit. If you miss a few times, it's okay—all is not lost. Don't give up. You'll get there.

Chapter Nine

July 2005

During the weeks before Cheryl's next appointment, she gave a lot of thought to working in additional meals, but even with her appointment looming, she still hadn't managed to get that second meal in before lunch. She never seemed to be organized enough to bring lunch into work. Just as predicted, by the time that midmorning hunger hit, she just didn't have time to order something, so she usually succumbed to junk food.

In spite of everything, though, Cheryl was still losing weight. When the scale brought yet another new low—228—Cheryl smiled and felt her determination intensify. She had to get that second morning meal in, but she just didn't know how to do it. Suddenly, she remembered Tina's offer to help. Until right then, Cheryl had forgotten Dr. Lang's suggestion of recruiting a co-worker to help. She could make arrangements with Tina to order lunch first thing in the morning.

The next morning, Cheryl took Tina aside and asked if she was still willing to help. Tina answered enthusiastically, "Sure! What do you want me to do?"

"Could you order me something for lunch now so that I have it by ten thirty? The doctor told me I should eat half of my lunch at that time."

"No problem—just tell me what to get."

"Cheryl, I need you in room three right now. Could you please drop whatever you're doing?" Dr. Weiner called out.

Cheryl dashed off to room three. "Surprise me," she called over her shoulder.

Tina had gotten lunch for Cheryl probably hundreds of times before, but Cheryl had always ordered what she wanted. Tina certainly knew what foods Cheryl liked, but they weren't exactly low in calories. As Cheryl handed an instrument to Dr. Weiner, she wondered what Tina would come up with.

At 10:40 Cheryl dashed up front to see if Tina had been able to get her anything. She was between patients, and her stomach was demanding its calories.

"Your sumptuous meal awaits you, m'lady," Tina said as she motioned with a flourish toward the conference room. Tina had laid out half a turkey club and an order of gazpacho. "I knew these items were low in calories," Tina said proudly. "I remembered that time we went to that Spanish restaurant on South Street, and you really liked the gazpacho. I hope this is okay—I hardly had time to order between all of those patients! I got Darlene to cover the phones while I picked it up."

"Thanks, Tina," Cheryl said, gazing at the unfamiliar meal in front of her and wondering if Tina had really done her a favor.

Cheryl was pleasantly surprised. The gazpacho wasn't quite as good as when she'd had it at Majorca, but it was still very palatable. By the time she had finished it, the half sandwich was almost more than she wanted. *This meal is certainly better than a bag of potato chips!* Tina hadn't ordered her anything to drink, so Cheryl had a glass of cold water. Remarkably, she actually liked the water better with the gazpacho than drinking a sweet soda. It took Cheryl only six and a half minutes to eat without interruption. Dr. Weiner was still on a phone call and hadn't yet started with the next patient. Cheryl had already set up the room; she hadn't missed a beat.

Cheryl finished up the morning hours in a very good mood. Even as the morning drew to a close, she still wasn't starving or imagining what food she was going to order. Lunchtime came before any real cravings did; she wasn't even all that hungry. When Tina produced the cucumber salad and the rest of the sandwich, Cheryl wasn't sure she wanted it at all. In fact, she ended up saving the last quarter of her sandwich for later. She drank water again. It wasn't bad.

As she was getting ready to leave work, Cheryl started to feel a bit hungry again and suddenly remembered her leftover club sandwich quarter. She ate it on the way to the bus, then chuckled to herself during the rest of the ride. Inadvertently, she had just had her fourth meal of the day. Granted, it wasn't the 350 calories it was supposed to be, but this was what Dr. Lang had been working her up to. She was almost home, and she was no longer very hungry.

That evening, Cheryl ate a salad with low-calorie ranch dressing along with her Lean Cuisine, and she was satisfied. She didn't want her mother's leftovers this time; she wrapped them up and decided to give them to her mom the following night.

Cheryl was curious. Today had been really satisfying ... and yet, she was quite sure that she had probably eaten far fewer calories than usual. Cheryl decided to look everything up in her calorie book and calculate the differences. She figured out one of her typical days: when she drank regular soda, it came to about 2,450 calories, but without the soda, it was 2,075. Amazingly, today she had eaten only 1,645—almost 400 calories less than one of her typical days without soda—and she felt good. It was hard to believe that the gazpacho was only sixty calories, and the cucumber salad only fifty. Even more unbelievable was the fact that she had really liked both. Maybe she was onto something.

She felt better about her upcoming appointment the next day, having finally worked out a way to get additional meals into her day. She wondered what the doctor wanted to discuss with her this time.

When Dr. Lang brought up the subject of exercise, Cheryl wasn't surprised at all. In fact, the sinking feeling in her stomach was far too familiar.

Uh-oh, Cheryl thought. She had known it was coming, but no way was she going to a gym and working out—no way.

"Is there any activity you enjoy doing that you might be able to squeeze into your schedule, such as tennis, volleyball, or even dancing?"

"I love to dance but have no one to dance with."

"What about taking lessons? From what I understand, dance studios don't just give lessons. They also have get-togethers, so you can find partners."

"I dunno. I'll think about it. Can I ask you a question? I mean, I know exercise is important—everyone talks about it—but can't I just lose the weight by eating less? Do I really have to exercise? I'm just so bad at it. I've tried before, and I've just never been able to do it for more than a few weeks. I get so bored."

"That's why I've suggested trying an activity that you like. And yes, exercise is very important. The reason you're trying to eat smaller, more frequent meals is to increase your metabolism. Exercise plays a huge role in increasing your metabolism. It determines how quickly or how slowly you lose weight. I'd like to discuss metabolism a little more without getting too technical so that you can have a better understanding of its importance. Remember that the more you know and understand about the process, the more apt you are to succeed. I don't want you to underestimate the importance of knowledge in any endeavor—especially this one!"

Cheryl nodded almost imperceptibly. She was very doubtful that exercise would become a habit. It never had worked before, and she was pretty certain that she didn't have what it took to make it work in the future. She tried very hard not to tune out as Dr. Lang's explanation droned on.

"As we discussed before, when we talk about metabolism in relation to weight loss, we're generically speaking about how quickly or slowly, or how efficiently or inefficiently, your body burns calories. Earlier, we talked about how eating more frequently throughout the day prevents the body from going into or staying in fasting mode, where it is working to conserve all its energy stores. Well, that's only one way to burn more calories. We already discussed how all the organs of your body burn energy just by going through their routine functions—your heart beating, your lungs breathing, and so on. And clearly, any average joe knows that exercise burns more calories. The more exercise you get, the more energy you burn, the more calories you use up, and the more the fat cells in your body shrink."

Cheryl agreed that exercise burned calories, but she always had known that. This scientific fact certainly wasn't going to change her reluctance to puff and sweat at the gym.

Dr. Lang continued. "Let me ask you this: are you puzzled by friends who are much thinner than you are despite eating more than you do?"

That question caught Cheryl's attention. "Isn't that because they eat more often, and their metabolism is faster?"

"That's only part of the reason. There's clearly an advantage to having never been overweight in the first place. If you've never lost and gained weight on a variety of occasions, then you'll have more muscle mass than someone who's been on that diet roller coaster. Do you know why that's important, and what it has to do with you?"

"Not really."

"I know that you know exercise is important. I am equally sure you realize that the more exercise you get, the more muscle you'll have, and the less exercise you get, the more that muscle atrophies or shrinks."

Cheryl's attention hadn't waned yet. She wanted to know why her friends had less trouble staying thin.

"What you may not realize," Dr. Lang continued, "is that the more muscle mass you have, the more calories you burn, even when you're not getting any exercise! This piece of information is necessary in understanding why people who have very different weights could still require the same amount of daily calories to sustain that same weight."

"So what you're saying is that someone who's thinner than I am may require the same amount of calories a day that I require, and will still stay thin?" Cheryl couldn't believe that some skinny person could eat exactly what she ate without gaining a pound. It didn't seem fair.

"That's exactly right. You see, for all intents and purposes, fat doesn't burn calories. Muscle does. The amount of muscle you have in your body, compared to the amount of fat, plays a large part in how many calories you burn each day, even when you're not doing anything."

"I know what I said is right, but I was really just parroting what you said to see if I was listening right. But I still don't understand how it works."

"Let me see if I can clarify it for you. The amount of calories you burn in a day, regardless of the amount of exercise, represents your basic metabolic rate. So if two people weighed exactly the same, but one person had 50 percent body fat while the other had only 20 percent body fat, the first person's basic metabolic rate would be quite different. The person with less fat and more muscle would require many more calories to maintain their body weight. They could then eat much more in a day than the person with more fat—without gaining a single ounce."

Cheryl still wasn't quite getting it.

Dr. Lang started writing on the exam table paper as she explained. "Let's say that Mary weighs 160 pounds, but she has 50 percent body fat and is five feet tall. Jane weighs 160 pounds, but only has 20 percent body fat, yet Jane is five foot ten inches tall. Mary's lean weight, without the fat, is 80 pounds—50 percent of 160. Jane's lean body weight is 128 pounds—80 percent of 160." Dr. Lang did the math: 100 percent - 20 percent body fat = 80 percent lean body mass.

"Since we burn approximately twelve and a half calories per pound of lean body weight, Mary's basic caloric requirement per day is 1,000 calories (remember, this includes no exercise whatsoever), and Jane's basic caloric requirement is 1,600 calories per day. If we postulate that each of them at the present time is only getting a moderate amount of exercise per day—moderate exercise burns about five calories per actual body weight pound—we would then add another 800 calories to their daily requirement. So in order to maintain their present weights, Mary can only have 1,800 calories per day to Jane's 2,400 calories per day. So there's Jane, eating up a storm—2,400 calories worth—without gaining an ounce, while poor Mary is only eating 1,800 calories per day and can't lose an ounce."

Dr. Lang looked up from the exam table. "Can you begin to see why the more fat content you have in your body, the more difficult it is to lose weight?"

"I think I'm getting it. People with more muscle burn more calories, and if I had more muscle in my body, I would burn more calories."

"Exactly."

"How can I find out how much body fat I have?"

"We can measure it. I'll go get the scale."

Dr. Lang had Cheryl stand on the special scale, then plugged in her age, weight, height, and the fact that she was female.

"Your body fat is 37 percent."

"What should it be?"

"The high end of normal for women is 27 percent."

"Gosh, how did mine get so high?"

"Believe it or not, dieting plays a role in increasing the percentage of body fat. Whenever you go on a diet and eat or absorb far fewer calories on a daily basis than your body requires, you not only lose fat, but you lose muscle as well. It's a generally accepted statistic that for every pound you lose on a scale, you lose approximately half a pound of fat and half a pound of muscle. Unfortunately, when you stop dieting and gain weight back, you primarily gain it back in the form of fat, not muscle—especially if you're not getting much exercise. So, every time you've been on a diet in the past, you've depleted your muscle mass and increased your body-fat percentage, making it more and more difficult to lose weight. If you have a good exercise program in place while losing and gaining weight, this might not occur as much. Unfortunately, the majority of patients I know hardly exercise at all."

At that moment, Cheryl wished she hadn't gone on all those diets.

Dr. Lang continued, "So now you are beginning to understand why, by necessity, changing your eating habits should be a slow process: not only because of the need for repetition over time to establish habits, but also because losing too much too fast can foil your efforts. You want to maintain muscle mass while losing fat. So now you can see why exercise is crucial."

Cheryl really was beginning to understand why exercise was so important. Maybe she would give dancing a try. She sure knew that going to a gym was out of the question. All the exercise equipment sitting in her basement gathering dust testified to her reluctance to use it ... and besides, she'd feel awkward as hell exercising in front of others.

Who would have thought I'd even be considering something like this? Cheryl thought. *I know I've just started, but I've come such a long way already!*

"I'd like to see you again in two months. That'll give you a chance to make some of the changes we've discussed in the past couple of weeks. Keep up the good work! And don't forget to pick up the chapter from my book on exercise."

"Oh, Dr. Lang, I almost forgot—my mother wanted me to ask you a question."

"Yes?"

"I was telling her that I needed to keep taking my medicine until my insulin levels were low again. She said that she was under the impression that when you have diabetes, your insulin levels are low, not high—and I guess so did I. So we're a little confused. Which is it?"

"It can be both. But usually, when the disease is caused by obesity, the levels are high. All juvenile diabetics and some adult-onset diabetics have insufficient insulin production. But in your case, your levels are too high, which means your pancreas is producing a lot of insulin, so that's a good thing ... but some of it is not working so well. Does that answer your question?"

"Yes—thank you, Doctor."

"My pleasure. Don't ever hesitate to ask me any questions. I'm always happy to answer them if I can. See you in two months."

Although Cheryl felt enthusiastic about the dancing idea when she left the office, by the time she'd gotten home, she was already having misgivings. If she didn't want to exercise in front of people, how could she learn to dance with others observing her? *Besides, who'd wanna dance with a tub o' lard like me?*

At dinner, Charlotte asked, "How'd it go at Dr. Lang's today?"

"All right, I guess." Cheryl responded reluctantly—she really was feeling anxious about exercising.

"But what else did she tell you to do?" Charlotte pressed.

"Well," Cheryl said with hesitation, "she told me I should think about exercise."

"Aha! Finally, something I understand. You gonna get all the exercise equipment you bought ages ago out of the basement?"

"No, Mom, and I'm not joining a gym. I already know myself well enough to not even bother with a membership I'll never use. She did suggest dancing, which you know I love, but I told her I had no partner to dance with. She suggested taking lessons at a dance studio—she said that I could find a partner there. I'm not sure I have the courage to go by myself, but maybe Teresa would be willing to go with me. I thought I'd give Teresa a call after dinner and ask her what she thought about the idea … that is, if I can find her home. Ever since she met this new guy, she's never around."

Charlotte looked skeptical. "Dancing as an exercise, huh? I don't know, kiddo. But any exercise has to be better than no exercise."

Cheryl cleaned up the kitchen and called Teresa when she was finished. Teresa answered on the second ring.

"Wow, you're actually home. So spill, girl: what's he like? I don't even know his name."

Cheryl heard what sounded like a sigh or a swoon over the phone. "His name is Michael—Michael Moreno. He's twenty-five. Never been married. He graduated from Penn State. He was there on a football scholarship—he wasn't good enough to go right to the pros, but he's just been drafted by the Eagles. He's a running back. He's not that big for a back, but to me, he's absolutely divine. You should see his abs … and oh, he's got the most amazing butt."

"Isn't he a little young, Teresa?"

"He acts really mature, and he has the most amazing body."

"Does he have anything upstairs? I mean these guys on football scholarships … aren't some of them really dumb?"

"He's not dumb. And did I tell you about his abs? It's a classic six-pack!"

Cheryl could see that her friend was majorly in lust, not love, but she wasn't going to rain on anyone's parade. All the same, she didn't think she'd see any wedding invitations any time soon. She breathed a selfish sigh of relief.

"So listen," Cheryl said cheerfully, "the reason I called was that I saw the doctor today, and she recommended I get some exercise doing something I enjoy. She suggested I take lessons at a dance studio. I'm not likely to do it by myself, so I was wondering if I could twist your arm to do it with me. It could be fun." She held her breath. If Teresa didn't want to do it, who would?

"Hey, that could be a really cool idea. Did you see that show *Dancing with the Stars?*"

Cheryl was taken aback. She hadn't expected such an enthusiastic response. "No, I didn't. Who was in it, and what kind of dancing did they do?"

"Several soap stars, actors, and even athletes teamed up with dance instructors. They competed in a contest with a bunch of different dances … I can't remember them all, but I know they talked about the rumba, the samba, and the tango. Oh, Cheryl, I wish you could have seen it—it was hilarious watching untrained actors and athletes struggling to learn to dance, but also inspiring when they did a really good job. I saw a news article saying that ever since the program began, ballroom dancing studios have been busier than ever."

Cheryl was really happy that Teresa was into the idea. "Do you know where we can find a dance studio?" Cheryl asked.

"Not a clue. But I'll look on the Internet and see if I can find one nearby. Great idea—I really think that could be a lot of fun. Listen, I'll call you tomorrow. Bye!"

"Bye." Cheryl was actually dumbfounded. Teresa had gotten her even more excited about the prospect. Her friend's enthusiasm was contagious. Maybe it would be fun.

Can you find ways to fit enjoyable exercise into your life?

STEP 5: GETTING EXERCISE AS PAINLESSLY AS POSSIBLE
By
Nikki Lang, MD

You knew before starting this book that exercise was important in your efforts to be slimmer, but you probably equated these beneficial results primarily with the extra calories you burned while exercising. Now you know that exercise plays a major role in maintaining and building muscle mass to help reduce your percentage of body fat.

But why does our muscle mass decline while our body fat increases? Well, obviously, the lack of planned exercise is a significant factor, but have you ever really considered how sedentary we've become in our everyday lives? Technology continues to make our lives easier, but has insidiously reduced our activity levels. If we can figure out how to make already required chores more active throughout the day *and* find ways to get additional planned exercise, we'll get much farther down the road of permanent weight control. This chapter will show you ways to do both.

It's really no secret that our society is made up of an increasing number of couch potatoes. We don't have to get up to answer the phone; we have our cordless or cell phones right next to us. We don't have to get up to change the channel on the TV; we have the remote control. Remember when we had to get out of the car to pull up the garage door? We often don't even bother to go shopping at the mall, instead sitting down at our computer and shopping online. Some of us don't even have to commute to work, since we work at home. Our society has become so physically lazy that when we do go shopping, we drive around for ten minutes in the parking lot, trying to find a spot close to the door so we don't have to walk too far. God forbid we would have to walk an extra fifty feet!

As each year goes by, we get less and less exercise, even during normal everyday activities. It's no wonder those tires are growing around our middles. In the beginning, I emphasized the importance of little changes and how they add up. Well, that works for exercise as well. Let's talk about what we can do every day, during a normal day, to work our muscles a little more.

From the examples above, you can surmise some of the simplest things to do. Return the cordless phone to its charging base when you aren't using it. Hide the TV remote so you have to get up to change the channel. Park at the back of the parking lot, away from other cars, so you have to walk farther to get to the door.

Do you have stairs in your house or apartment? Do you put things on the stairs so that you can take them up when you're on your way up anyway? Instead, each time you have something to take upstairs, do it right then.

Do you work in an office building? Walk up the stairs every day instead of taking the elevator. "But I work on the sixteenth floor!" you might say. In that case, take the elevator to the fourteenth floor and walk up the last two flights. When you get less winded walking up two flights, start getting off at the thirteenth floor. You get the picture. I've seen people wait at the hospital for an elevator to go to the second floor for as long as seven minutes, when walking to the second floor would have taken less than a minute.

Throughout your day, if you keep your mind attentive, you can find opportunities to get a little extra exercise—sometimes in the most unlikely places. In the morning when you brush your teeth, you probably have to bend over the sink. Well, instead of bending from the waist, why not bend from the knees to get closer to the sink? Give those thighs a little workout.

How about when you need to get something out of a bottom drawer? Squat down instead of bending over. Need to pick something up? Squat and lift; we all know it's better for our backs anyway. When you find yourself halfway down a flight of stairs, walk back up and then back down again. It will only take you another ten to twenty seconds, but that's good exercise. All of these little workouts will add up.

But what about more vigorous exercise? It's easy for me to tell you to join a gym and exercise regularly, and if you have the discipline and fortitude to do so, that plan will work great. I suspect, however, that you've tried that in the past, and it hasn't worked out very well. Your intentions were always very good, but the time you spent in the gym dwindled to nothing, and you're still kicking yourself for that one-year membership you wasted. Or perhaps several pieces of exercise equipment are now sitting in a corner somewhere, gathering dust or serving as clothing trees. Either way, you know the drill: such exercise is dull and tough to stick with.

How can you avoid lost gym memberships and dusty exercise equipment? If you can find physical activities you look forward to doing, rather than dreading, your chances of turning exercise into a habit improve considerably.

I'd like to tell you about one of my most successful patients. This patient—let's call him Sam—weighed about 285 pounds. He had come into the office for a physical and routine blood work and was found to be diabetic with a rather high cholesterol level and mild hypertension. He took my healthy eating advice very seriously and lost significant amounts of weight over the next year. Even more important, he began to exercise. He had always loved to play ice hockey, but had been so out of shape that he had not done so for quite a while. When he realized that exercise was important, he joined an amateur league in his neighborhood. After a while, he was playing ice hockey at least three times a week—sometimes more. Now that's what I call exercise!

Approximately a year and a half later, I saw him for some minor problem. He then weighed 185 pounds, and he proudly showed me his stomach, which was hard as a rock. He felt great. Not only that, his blood pressure and sugar were normal. His cholesterol was much improved as well.

Why do I relate this story? Because Sam found a form of exercise that he loved. He didn't have to force himself to go to the gym. He couldn't wait to get back to the hockey rink and *play* some more. If you can find some form of exercise that you enjoy, you'll actually look forward to doing it. Obviously, if you can participate in some sport with friends or acquaintances by joining a volleyball league or a softball league or taking up tennis, you can get your exercise and have some fun at the same time. Suppose you're not athletic? You can take swing dance, square dance, or even salsa lessons.

Meet other people and learn to do something fun after work that will help you unwind—and help you get some exercise. If you're shy, bring a friend. If you can't seem to find an activity that excites you, then perhaps your group of friends can try something more simple, yet social, like power walking. Maybe the enjoyable conversation will help you stick with it.

Brainstorm with family and friends. What activities can you do together? Try playing hopscotch with the kids or jumping rope. Twister is a game that can be played indoors. These activities can become contests; whoever loses has to cook dinner or do some other housekeeping chore that he or she doesn't ordinarily do.

Make up your own games or contests, as long as some exercise comes out of it. Who can walk the longest on their heels without letting their toes touch the ground? Who can walk the fastest on their toes, keeping one foot touching the ground at all times? Who can stand on one leg the longest? A three-legged race only requires four people. Keep track of each person's points for the week, declaring a winner at the end of each one.

Make sure you all agree on a reward before the contest begins. Remember, you're trying to form a new habit. So make sure you establish a set time, several times a week, to have your contest. It doesn't have to take more than ten minutes and can be a fun family activity.

You'll notice a bigger difference in your body and experience a new level of success if you're willing to find creative ways to incorporate exercise into your daily life.

Let's review our steps.

Step 1: Stop drinking your calories

Step 2: Eat breakfast

Step 3: Eat a small meal between breakfast and lunch

Step 4: Eat an appetizer a few hours before dinner

Step 5: Find exercise that you enjoy.

Chapter Ten

July 2005

Teresa called Cheryl on her cell phone on the way to work. "You won't believe this," Teresa said, her voice full of excitement, "but a new dance studio just opened at Headhouse Square. It's just a few blocks from work for both of us. Well, actually I don't think it's new, I just hadn't noticed it before. But isn't that cool? We could go after work. What d'ya think?"

"That sounds great ... but I don't know. I can't really go right after work. I mean, I have to go home and get dinner for my mom and ... and I'm not sure I want to go after work," Cheryl finished lamely. She was getting cold feet. Did she really want to do this?

"Couldn't you get Mrs. Curtis or Mrs. O'Hara to sort out your mom's dinner one day of the week?"

Cheryl was pretty sure she could; her anxiety was the issue. Yes, she loved to dance at parties and weddings, but she had never tried structured dancing. She was beginning to wonder if she could learn those fancy dances with those tricky steps. Besides, she'd watched some ballroom dancing in a movie years ago—what was the name of it? Oh, yeah, *Strictly Ballroom*. The man would fling the lady and make her dip. *That's a laugh—I'd be flat on the floor in no time.* She didn't want to be laughed at.

"I'm not sure if I could ... I'll have to ask them," she answered hesitantly. "I'll call you later tonight." As she hung up the phone, she felt guilty that she had involved Teresa and gotten her excited, only to let her friend down.

She didn't call Teresa back, nor did she mention the dancing lessons to her mom, nor did she ask Mrs. Curtis or Mrs. O'Hara if they could see to her mom's dinner once a week. She just didn't want to be put in a position to be made fun of.

She didn't hear from Teresa for almost a week. She guessed that Michael, with the great abs, was at the top of Teresa's agenda. That was fine with Cheryl. She had convinced herself that dancing lessons were the last thing she wanted to do. No way was she going to make a fool of herself.

On Friday night, Cheryl and her mom were just finishing dinner when Charlotte asked, "So, are you going dancing tonight?"

"What gave you that idea?" Cheryl queried.

"Last week, you told me you were going to take dancing lessons if Teresa was okay with it … and you told me she wasn't only okay with it, but was really excited by the idea. So I just assumed you'd be going."

"Well, I just … just decided that I didn't want to. I didn't want to leave you alone too much."

"Cheryl Morris, don't you go blaming me, young lady. That's the feeblest excuse I've ever heard!"

"No, really, Mom. There's a dance studio just a few blocks from work, but that would mean I wouldn't be coming home after work, and on top of that, I wouldn't get in 'til late. Who would get you dinner and make sure you took your pills?"

"I repeat: that is the feeblest excuse I've ever heard. Don't use me to hide behind. You know very well that Mollie Curtis or Maggie O'Hara would be more than willing to help out. What's stopping you? I know it's not me."

"Nothing's stopping me, Ma."

"You know I can't stand to be lied to. So when you're done telling fibs, I'll talk to you again." With that, Charlotte pushed herself away from the table and wheeled herself into the living room to watch TV.

Cheryl never could put anything over on her mother, and now her mother was angry with her; Cheryl hated that. She tiptoed around her mother all evening, not saying a word. When Cheryl passed by Charlotte to go into the kitchen, she asked her mother politely if she could get her anything. Her mother didn't answer.

At about her mother's usual bedtime, Cheryl tried to push Charlotte's wheel-chair into the bedroom. Charlotte had set the brake on her wheelchair and wouldn't let Cheryl release it. She remained stone silent.

"Okay, Mom, you win!" Cheryl finally exclaimed. "I'm afraid I'll make a fool of myself. That's why I don't want to do it. I'm too big for all that fancy dancing stuff. If somebody tries to dip me back, we'll both end up on the floor. Who could possibly hold me up? I doubt any weight lifter would be graceful enough to be a dance instructor. There—you satisfied now?"

"Well, I knew I wasn't the reason, but I still don't understand. But why do you think people will laugh at you? You've always been such a good dancer. I doubt anyone with half a brain would try to teach you anything that would be physically impossible. I know how much you hate getting out of your comfort zone, but honey, Teresa's right: it probably would be fun. This is a great way to get that exercise." Charlotte started coughing and wheezing. That was probably the longest sentence she'd spoken in ages. She didn't have quite enough air to finish the last few words, which came out something like "exxxxxerrrrchise."

Her mom was right: Cheryl was letting her imagination get too far ahead of her. What 150-pound guy was going to try to hold her up? He wouldn't want to look foolish any more than she did.

"You're right, Mom. You're such a wise old witch," she said affectionately. "I'll call Teresa tomorrow." This time, Charlotte let her daughter release the brake and wheel her to her bedroom. Cheryl tucked her into bed and kissed her on her forehead. "I love you, Mom. I know you just want me to be happy. I'm trying, I really am."

The doctor said a lot of different kinds of changes needed to be made, Cheryl remembered as she watched her mother fall asleep. She was only beginning to realize how many.

As promised, Cheryl called Teresa the next day.

"So," Teresa said, "you were going to get back to me about the dancing lessons. What gives?"

"Sorry. To tell the truth, I was getting cold feet … but yes, I've sorted out some free time after work. Why don't we meet up tomorrow at the dance studio and find out more about how it works?"

"Super!" Teresa was delighted.

Cheryl couldn't wait to tell her friend about her progress and how few calories she had eaten without really trying.

"So maybe this doctor really knows what she's talking about," Teresa mused. "Maybe it really is about an attitude."

"I'm beginning to believe." Cheryl knew she hadn't sounded so optimistic in a long time.

"Well, I'm very happy for you, and I can't wait to go dancing. So I'll see you tomorrow at the dance studio after work?"

"Absolutely," Cheryl answered, smiling on her end.

Teresa signed off with "Ciao," and hung up.

Cheryl stared at the receiver. *Ciao?* That Italian football player was really getting under Teresa's skin. *Whatever,* she thought, *as long as she meets me at the dance studio tomorrow.*

The next evening found Cheryl pacing up and down the sidewalk in front of the Society Hill Dance Studio, glancing at her watch every few minutes. *Where was Teresa? She should've been here by now.* It was almost six. She made up her mind that if Teresa didn't show in the next five minutes, she was gone. People were coming and going from the studio, and although it might have been her imagination, they seemed to be looking at her in a way that said, "What's a fat girl like you doing in a place like this?" None of the people she saw looked like her—they looked slender, graceful. *I don't belong here*, Cheryl thought dismally.

Teresa arrived in the nick of time, breathless. She had practically run all the way from the store. One of her salespeople—the one who was designated to stay for the evening and lock up later—had gone out to get a bite to eat and lost track of the time. Teresa apologized profusely to Cheryl. "Come on, let's go in," Teresa said as she grabbed Cheryl by the hand, practically dragging her up the steps. Cheryl followed reluctantly.

They entered a large room, unadorned save for the very large rectangular mirrored columns in the middle. Students and instructors danced in multiple corners and alcoves of the room. *This place must have an interesting sound system*, Cheryl thought. Everyone appeared to be dancing to different rhythms.

The reception desk—or rather, counter—was just to their left and slightly behind them. They had nearly walked right past it. A blonde woman, very pleasant looking and of indeterminate age, stood behind the counter, talking on the phone. She was flipping through a loose-leaf notebook, apparently trying to schedule someone for an appointment with one of the studio's private instructors. When the woman saw Cheryl and Teresa, she motioned to them to come over, then stuck a finger in the air, mouthing that she'd be with them in just a minute.

After hanging up the phone, she turned to them with a smile. "Sorry about that. Can I help you?"

"We'd like to find out about dancing lessons," Teresa answered.

"You've certainly come to the right place. What we usually suggest is for you to take a private class first—which, by the way, is absolutely free. During that time, you tell the instructor what type of dances you're interested in learning, and he has an opportunity to evaluate your ability. Then you can continue with private lessons or choose from an array of group lessons. He will then assist with your selections to make sure you're in the right group."

"Can we do our class together?" Cheryl asked nervously, gesturing to Teresa. She didn't want to do it by herself.

"Sure, no problem," the receptionist replied. "Every Tuesday, we also have an open house dance party. This gives all our students an opportunity to practice their skills. If you look just behind you and to the left"—the girls glanced around and saw a shelf—"there are a number of flyers that have a lot of the information you'll need."

Cheryl and Teresa walked over to get a closer look. One flyer advertised a class for "wedding preparation."

"Harvey and Susan sure could have used these lessons," Teresa said, barely containing her laughter.

Suddenly, they both burst out in hysterics, remembering Susan and Harvey's first dance together as a wedding couple. Harvey just didn't dance, but he had tried very hard to comply with Susan's wishes for just this one dance. On his third step, he had trod on her dress, lost his balance, and knocked Susan to the floor. In his attempts not to fall on top of her, he managed to jump over her and hold himself up for a few more unbalanced steps, finally landing on the nearest table. He knocked over the centerpiece, throwing flowers and water all over his boss's wife. She was not impressed. Harvey had yet to live that day down. Needless to say, he never danced again, much to Susan's disappointment.

"Do you really think lessons would've helped? Even if he hadn't stepped on her dress?" Cheryl struggled to stop laughing. "He looked like a robot with its batteries running down."

Cheryl felt so much more relaxed. She couldn't remember the last time she had laughed so hard. She was finally ready to schedule her first lesson. She walked back over to the reception area, with Teresa following. After some difficulty coordinating everyone's schedules, Teresa and Cheryl finally settled on Friday at six thirty. Cheryl would have to check with Mrs. Curtis and make sure she could stay after the bridge game to take care of her mom for dinner. She knew her mother wouldn't eat unless someone set a plate of the food in front of her, and Charlotte couldn't afford not to eat.

Their instructor's name was Victor. The receptionist said he was a very good dancer who had won a number of dance competitions. "Even better for beginners like you, he's an excellent teacher," she added. "You girls are going to have a great time!"

Cheryl was pretty hungry by the time she got home. Unlike the other day, when she had eaten the last quarter of her club sandwich after work, she'd had nothing for the end of the day. Tina had tried to duplicate her previous success in ordering food for Cheryl, choosing vegetable soup, a tuna fish sandwich, and a three-bean salad. But Cheryl hated the vegetable soup, so she just ate half the tuna sandwich. At lunchtime, she was pretty hungry. She tried to eat the three-bean salad, but after one or two bites, she gave up—not her cup of tea. So, all she had eaten was the other half of her tuna fish sandwich. She'd had nothing left over to eat later in the day. On top of that, she was still hungry after the tuna sandwich, and as a result had succumbed to a bag of chips as well as two chocolate-chip cookies.

She pulled out her mom's leftover dinner from the previous night, then added two more Lean Cuisines. She was hungry. She gave her mom the leftovers and ate two whole dinners herself. Not the most successful day in the eating department, but she had a dance lesson scheduled for Friday. She was determined to focus on her successes and work harder in preventing her failures.

Cheryl knew she couldn't blame Tina for the food choices and had to take more responsibility in choosing her menu. She brought home a copy of the deli takeout menu to study, then circled the foods she liked so that Tina would have a better chance at ordering for her appropriately.

She mulled over the conversation she planned to have with Tina in the morning, wanting to tell her how much she appreciated her help and to make sure Tina wasn't mad at her for not eating everything that she ordered. Having only just gotten started on her journey, Cheryl knew better than anyone how very long it was going to be, and she would need all the help she could get.

Six pounds down, eighty-four to go!

Chapter Eleven

July 2005

Over the following week, since visiting the dance studio, Teresa and Cheryl had been making plans on the phone almost nightly. They both decided that they wanted to take lessons in swing dancing. Cheryl already knew how to swing dance. Teresa said she didn't think she was all that good at it, but she loved it too.

Teresa was, however, particularly enthusiastic about taking samba lessons as well. She thought it was a really sexy dance and loved Brazilian samba music. One of her favorite songs was "The Girl from Ipanema." Cheryl wasn't so sure about the samba. She, too, liked the music, but she thought it required a lot of hip action and wasn't so sure she would be able to get her hips going like that. And besides, who could see her hips anyway? She thought a dance that was more about the steps, like the Argentine tango—or maybe even the cha-cha—would be better for her.

Neither of them was interested in the waltz, but Teresa brought up the possibility of the two-step.

"What's the two-step?" Cheryl asked.

"I can't really explain it," said Teresa, "but I saw them do it on *Dancing with the Stars*, and I kind of liked it. It was sort of like the waltz in the way you move across the floor with your partner, but it's much faster, and you have to use your feet more. Actually, I'm not really sure I know what I'm talking about, but I sure liked the way John O'Hurley and his partner did it. It's kind of sophisticated, but at the same time really energetic, and if you're doing this to get exercise, I think we should make sure we pick dances that require a bit of action. Don't you?"

"Well, of course—that makes sense. Maybe we should wait until our lesson and collaborate a little more with the instructor about the best course of action."

"That's fine with me. Did you get everything squared away with Mrs. Curtis for Friday night?"

"Yup, everything's a go," said Cheryl. "You know, I'm really kind of looking forward to this. I hope we like our instructor."

"Yeah, me too. Sometimes that can be half the battle. Maybe if it's a really good experience, I'll drag Michael there. That would be so cool if we could dance well together—especially something like the samba."

"That would be sweet to have a boyfriend who could dance well. Do you think Michael would be willing to take lessons?" Cheryl asked, fearful that Teresa might end up taking lessons with him and not herself.

"I think he might be willing, but I'm not sure he'd be able to find the time," Teresa answered with a sigh.

Cheryl was relieved. "Not to change the subject, but do you want to grab some dinner before the lesson, or should we eat afterward?"

"I think we should go afterward," Teresa answered. "We won't be pressed for time then, and we could maybe treat ourselves to a nice dinner. Maybe at Gnocchi? They have great Italian food, and it's really reasonably priced. Michael took me there one night. I was impressed."

"Sold," said Cheryl, recognizing she was beginning to feel ever so slightly jealous of Michael. "So, I'll see you at the dance studio on Friday at six thirty."

"Looking forward to it … ciao." And with that, Teresa was no longer there. Cheryl found herself staring again at a silent receiver.

Cheryl was both excited for and afraid of the dance lesson. When she had said that she hoped they liked the instructor, she was really more anxious about the instructor's ability to set her at ease, despite her body type. She really did love to dance.

Cheryl was so busy all week that Friday came upon her sooner than expected. She was almost out the door Friday morning when she suddenly realized that she should take some shoes to change into for dancing. The sneakers she wore for work wouldn't do well on a dance floor. She picked up shoe after shoe, tossing each pair over her shoulder in disgust. She wanted something that would slide on the dance floor, but would also be comfortable. She didn't want to wear heels, because by the time she finished the lesson, she would be wincing with every step. She couldn't make up her mind, so she threw several pairs into a gym bag. Her instructor could help her make the choice.

She ran out the door a little late, but what else was new?

The day went smoothly. She had gone over the menu with Tina earlier in the week, and that had paid off. She was now eating a midmorning meal a few hours before lunch, and usually had a little something for the end of the day. She hadn't yet sorted out the calorie counts, but she had a feeling that they weren't far from the 300–350 calories that Dr. Lang had suggested. Cheryl had been teased a bit with questions about what was in her gym bag, but she refused to share.

The last patient ran a little bit late, but that was fine with Cheryl, since she would have a little time to kill before her lesson. In spite of staying late at work, she still arrived at the studio a few minutes early.

Cheryl watched another dancer taking a lesson. She wasn't very good. The instructor had to keep going over and over the same step. The student was pretty and thin, but she clearly didn't know how to dance. *Looks like she's gonna need that fifty-class package.* Cheryl felt more relaxed. Someone else didn't know what she was doing either.

Teresa finally arrived at 6:25, and they went to the reception desk. "Do you have an appointment?" the receptionist asked.

"Yes," they chimed in simultaneously.

"And who is your instructor?"

"Victor." This time it was just Teresa that answered.

"Just a second, and I'll get him for you." She checked her scheduling book as she said it, and within seconds, she slipped from behind the desk and disappeared.

She returned minutes later with Victor by her side. As he walked toward them, Cheryl's heart skipped a beat. He was tall, dark, and handsome. And in spite of his height, he looked to her like the spitting image of Al Pacino, with his olive complexion and his brooding eyes. His casual but stylish shirt and trousers gave Cheryl the impression that he had just walked off a photo shoot set at *Esquire* magazine.

"Good evening, ladies. How are you tonight?"

"Anxious to get started," replied Teresa. Cheryl said nothing. Her tongue was glued to the inside of her mouth.

Victor went around behind the reception counter and pulled out two clipboards with some blank information sheets on them. "If you don't mind, could you please complete these forms so I can get a better idea of what brought you here?"

They took the forms and quickly completed them. It was just the usual demographic information—name, address, and so on. The form included two lists to check off. One listed the types of dances clients might be interested in, and the second requested the reasons a customer wanted to take lessons. Cheryl checked the box next to "health reasons." Teresa marked the one for fun.

Victor perused the two clipboards with an efficient glance. "I see here, Teresa, that you're interested in both swing and samba; and you, Cheryl, are also interested in swing, but would like to try the tango." He made no mention of why they were taking lessons. This made Cheryl a little more comfortable.

"So why don't we start with a few basic swing steps, since you'll be taking this lesson together? You can decide later if you want to take separate classes for either the tango or the samba. I'll help you with that decision."

"That would be great," Teresa responded.

Cheryl remained tongue-tied. She managed to nod, though.

Having settled on swing dancing for the moment, Victor indicated they should get started on their lesson. "Follow me, ladies." Victor led them to a corner of the dance studio around a small wall behind the reception desk. "You can put your belongings on one of those chairs. Okay, who wants to be first?"

Teresa volunteered, so Victor took her right hand in his left and placed her left hand on his shoulder. They remained a foot or so apart, but one could see that he was holding her firmly as he explained the basic steps and gestured for her to follow. Teresa did this awkwardly at first, but after a few repetitions, she seemed to catch on.

"Okay, Teresa, why don't you have a seat, and let's have Cheryl give it a try." Cheryl had still said absolutely nothing. Victor allowed her the silence, almost as though he sensed her nervousness. He simply took her hand and assumed the same position he had with Teresa. He then re-explained what they were about to do. Cheryl had observed his dancing with Teresa very carefully, and with her previous experience, she followed the first time without a single misstep. "That was excellent, Cheryl. Why don't we try the next few steps?" Again, Cheryl caught on quickly. She was very pleased with herself.

Victor asked Cheryl to sit out while he taught Teresa the next few steps. It was a tedious chore. Teresa was slow at picking up the newer steps, which had to be repeated over and over again. Cheryl was getting frustrated. She wanted her turn again; she liked it when Victor was touching her.

Finally, Teresa sat and Victor invited Cheryl to dance again. Cheryl wouldn't have minded spending the rest of the evening in his arms, but the lesson was just about over. The fifty minutes had whizzed by. Victor brought the lesson to a very abrupt end by sitting down with them to discuss the intricacies of the various dance courses and the costs of the private lessons—noting discounts they could get if they bought various combination packages. Cheryl still hadn't said a single word.

When he discussed which classes the women should take, Cheryl could tell he was being very careful not to hurt Teresa's feelings. He suggested that Teresa might want to take a beginner's class in swing, while Cheryl might benefit more from the advanced class. Of course, they could continue to take private lessons; in spite of their differences, he felt he could still teach them both, with Teresa benefiting from watching Cheryl.

Finally, Cheryl opened her mouth and said very quietly, "You know, I'm taking these lessons to try and get some exercise. I was wondering what dances you think would be the best for helping me to lose weight. You know—which one would make me work the hardest?"

"Well," said Victor, "swing is a very good choice, but if you really want to burn calories, I would suggest the salsa. It will really get your heart going, and many of the more complicated steps could be practiced at home, giving you even more exercise." Cheryl immediately clammed up again, but she managed a grateful smile. Teresa thanked him for his time, while Cheryl nodded in agreement.

"We'll be in touch when we figure out what we want to do," Teresa said with finality in her voice.

"Good evening, ladies." Victor bowed ever so slightly, and with that, turned to move on to his next lesson.

As they left the studio, Cheryl's mouth accelerated from zero to fifty during the two steps it took to get out the door. "Oh, my! Wasn't he adorable? He looks just like Al Pacino, except he's much taller. Oh, my … he was so cute. I couldn't stop looking at him. I'm surprised I didn't step all over my own feet, I was so nervous. For a second there, I thought I was going to puke right in his face. I can't believe how nervous I was. Teresa, don't you think he was absolutely gorgeous?"

"Are you serious?" Teresa asked, clearly baffled. "Do you really think he looked like Al Pacino? I mean maybe the nose and his complexion are similar, but Al Pacino … I don't think so."

"I can't believe you don't see it. Well, in a way, I'm glad—at least you won't be interested in him. Not that I think he'll ever be interested in me anyway, but at least I can fantasize about him. It's been ages since I've even done that."

They began discussing the lesson itself, but arrived at the restaurant before they could finish. It was a little crowded, but one or two small tables were still available, so the women were seated immediately. Cheryl looked around.

"This place has a really nice atmosphere. I like it," Cheryl remarked. She saw that many of the customers had brought their own bottles of wine. The restaurant was a BYOB, as were many of the small eateries in Philly. She and Teresa hadn't really thought about that, but neither of them drank very much alcohol anyway. She thought about coming here one night with Victor on a date. Sure, that was wishful thinking. But as she had said before, she was allowed to fantasize, wasn't she?

"So what do you want to eat?" Teresa asked.

Cheryl hadn't even looked at the menu. When she did, she was surprised at how reasonable it was. "I really don't know. Do you have any good ideas?"

"Well, the last time I was here, I had the chicken marsala, which was very good. I would recommend that. I think I'll have the chicken again, but I think this time I'll try the picante. Are you going to get an appetizer?"

"No, actually, I'm not that hungry … but I do think I will get the marsala. It sounds good."

They ordered their food and a bottle of water. Cheryl was actually beginning to prefer water to soda with a meal. Somehow, it just tasted better to her … strange.

"So what do you think about the salsa idea?" Teresa asked.

"It sounds pretty good to me," Cheryl replied. "I like the idea of practicing dance steps on my own, and from what I know of the swing, most of the more difficult parts almost always seem to require a partner. Besides, I really like the idea of learning something totally new. What about you? It's not the samba, but as I recall, it can still be a fairly sexy dance."

"Yeah, it is kind of appealing," Teresa continued, "and I really do like that kind of music. The rhythm instruments make it so you can hardly sit still. I remember, not too long ago, passing by a salsa band playing outdoors someplace in South Philly. I don't remember where, but as I was walking by, I couldn't help moving in step with the music. It really is infectious. I'm not a very good dancer, though. I hope I can learn it."

"Then salsa it is! Should we take private lessons or sign up for a group? I don't know about you, but I'd like to take a few private lessons first before making a fool of myself in front of a lot of other people." Cheryl crossed her fingers under the table. She really wanted to take some more private lessons with Victor, but she needed to convince Teresa. She wouldn't quite have the nerve to sign up by herself.

"I don't know." Teresa hesitated. "It really is a bit expensive. I mean, ninety dollars a week for a single private lesson? That's a lot of money."

"But we'll be splitting the cost, so it'll only be forty-five," Cheryl argued.

"Let me think about it," Teresa responded.

Dinner arrived. They ate without much further discussion. Cheryl thoroughly enjoyed her chicken marsala, wishing she could cook chicken this good. She ate the greens, but only ate one or two of the gnocchi that came with the dinner. They were a little mushy for her liking. She'd never had them before but decided she probably wouldn't again. The chicken was a rather generous portion, so she asked for a doggie bag. *I don't think I've ever done this before*, she thought in wonder as her server handed her the bag.

All in all, Cheryl thought the day had been very successful. She looked forward to seeing Victor again, but she wasn't going to pressure Teresa for an answer. She'd wait a few days, hoping he'd still have some openings next Friday.

Chapter Twelve

August 2005

The next month or so passed rather quickly. Teresa decided to go ahead and take the private lessons, thrilling Cheryl. Teresa still didn't catch on nearly as quickly as Cheryl, but at least they had both started at the same place: neither of them knew anything about salsa dancing. Cheryl still remained mostly mute during the classes, but after the women left the studio, her mouth would run like a motor. They continued to eat dinner at Gnocchi after each lesson. Cheryl made doggy bags a routine. She really liked the leftovers.

Cheryl was still bringing her gym bag to work, arousing the continued curiosity of her co-workers. Only now, the bag contained a special pair of shoes that she had purchased at Teresa's store—but only after much prodding. They were a bit expensive, but they were made of really soft Italian leather. They were blissfully comfortable and perfect for dancing. Cheryl often disappeared into her room right after dinner, and the sound of Latin music usually wasn't far behind. The full-length mirror hanging on the back of Cheryl's door showed a better dancer every week as Cheryl practiced her newest dance steps over and over again until they were perfect. She wanted Victor to be impressed; it was apparent even to Cheryl that he enjoyed dancing with her.

In addition to the improvements in her dancing, Cheryl was pleased at the amount of exercise she was getting. Sometimes she would perspire so much just from practicing that she'd have to take a shower before she went to bed.

Tomorrow marked her fifth appointment with Dr. Lang, and Cheryl was again looking forward to it. She couldn't believe the changes she had made in her life in just four short months. She was exercising almost on a daily basis and looking forward to her beloved dancing, even when her plans for the night included only practicing. She loved the music and the rhythm, and her progress made her feel good about herself. In spite of her weight, she was light on her feet.

Most days, she was eating five small meals. Cheryl couldn't believe how little junk food she was eating. She hadn't had one regular soda or fruit juice and was starting to drink a lot more water. True to her promise to her mom, she hadn't had one Snickers bar. She was pretty sure her mom had kept up her side of the bargain as well; Cheryl hadn't smelled cigarette smoke in the house for at least three months.

Cheryl couldn't wait to see what Dr. Lang had to say. She had lost an additional ten pounds since her last visit, setting her new low at 221. More amazing still, it hadn't been that hard. Well, yes, giving up the soda and the sugar and getting started on the dance lessons had been challenging, but not that hard, thanks to the help and support of her friends. Like Dr. Lang said, changes were difficult. But Cheryl wasn't walking around hungry and feeling deprived.

Cheryl was truly beginning to understand what it was about. These changes were really beginning to become habits. Oh, she wasn't going to be complacent about it and risk a soda or a Snickers bar, but she could see what was happening. She was starting to have confidence that if she could just stay on the same track, not only might she lose some more weight, but she also could even be thin again.

Cheryl arrived early again at the doctor's office. While she was waiting in the reception area, she thought about yet another new habit that had formed. Previously, she would arrive a little late at most places, but these days, she was on time or even early. She wondered what that meant psychologically, surely some hidden meaning had escaped her. But before she had any more time to ponder, Latisha called her back.

Sure enough, Cheryl had lost an additional ten pounds. Not only that, but her blood pressure was 128/78, the lowest she could remember for a long time. Needless to say, she still had to be measured with the larger cuff, but it didn't bother her so much. She was too busy feeling pleased with her new blood pressure.

Dr. Lang was very pleased also, and told her so. "Has it been that difficult?" she asked Cheryl.

"Actually, no. You were right: it does get easier. And I'm starting to see where forming habits is really key to the process."

"Are you getting any exercise?"

"Oh, yes! I'm taking salsa dancing lessons weekly, and boy, does that make you sweat! And I practice almost every night."

"Excellent, Cheryl. I can't tell you how gratifying it is to see you doing so well. I meet with so many patients, and it's always such a pleasure when someone gets it. So, are you ready to move on?"

"I really am," Cheryl answered enthusiastically.

"First of all, how are you doing with keeping your meals within the 300–350 calorie range?"

"Sometimes better than others. I order a lot of food out, and even splitting lunch in half puts me way over for each meal. But a lot of times, it's right on target. I don't look up everything I eat, but when I do, I realize that sometimes I'm eating much better than at other times without even knowing it."

"Have you figured out what the differences are in any of those meals you've looked up?"

"Well, of course, fast foods are ridiculously high for what you get. I mean a tiny little sausage-and-egg sandwich from McDonalds is 550 calories. If I tried to eat only 350 calories' worth, I'd have to get rid of almost a third of the sandwich, and it's a tiny little sandwich to start with."

"Exactly," said Dr. Lang. "So what makes the difference between a satisfying meal that's only 350 calories and one that isn't?"

"I'm not sure. I mean, I know when I have gazpacho along with only half a sandwich, I find that more satisfying, and the gazpacho only has only sixty calories."

"You're absolutely on the right track. We are satisfied by the volume of the food that we eat, not by the calories. So the more low-density foods we eat, the larger the volume, and the fewer the calories we consume. Can you figure out what I mean by 'low-density foods'?"

"Mmmm … vegetables?"

"Right—vegetables and fruits. Vegetables and fruits have very high water and fiber content. Since we don't digest most fiber, and water has no calories, most vegetables and fruits are very low in calories for the amount of volume they provide. A cup of lettuce has about 10 calories, and a cup of cheddar cheese has about 800 calories. I'd like to give you another chapter from my book that explains all of this in more depth, because I want to discuss one other idea with you."

"What's that?"

"I'd like you to learn how to cook."

"Whoa, wait a minute! I'm a disaster in the kitchen. I don't know the first thing about cooking … and anyway, why should that be important?"

"It's more important than you think. Being able to cook allows you to have much greater variety in your meals. Knowing what goes into the foods you're eating helps you distinguish why you like or dislike certain foods and teaches you how to make something boring into something far more interesting. A piece of chicken breast stuck in a broiler for a few minutes, without seasoning, can be awfully dry and uninteresting, but seasoned properly, or with the right sauce, it can be absolutely delicious."

Cheryl thought of her chicken marsala. She could learn how to make chicken marsala.

"Vegetables are so very important to the process of healthy eating," Dr. Lang continued, "and learning to prepare them according to your palate requires that you know some of the necessary subtleties of cooking."

"I'm not so sure," Cheryl resisted.

"Let me ask you a question. You often eat Lean Cuisines, right?"

"I do. They really help me out a lot, since the calorie count is so good."

"So tell me. Do you always like the vegetables they give you?"

"No. Sometimes they're really disgusting—all soggy and everything!"

"So then what do you do?" Dr. Lang asked.

"I don't eat them."

"So, are you then satisfied with your meal, or do you look for something else to eat?"

"I usually eat what my mom hasn't eaten ... or yeah, I'll root around in the kitchen for something else."

"My point exactly. If you had a generous helping of vegetables that you liked, that wouldn't happen so often."

"I've tried buying more vegetables, but they always end up rotting in my salad drawer."

"Buy fresh frozen vegetables. I find they're often fresher than the ones you buy at the market. I'm sure some people would disagree with me, but in my experience, fresh vegetables are often already days old by the time they've been shipped and displayed. Who knows how long they've been sitting on the supermarket shelf? Frozen vegetables, on the other hand, are frozen right after they're picked. If you buy frozen, you don't have to worry about them rotting in your refrigerator. Buy them in bags, then take as little or as much as you want at a time, and put the rest back in the freezer.

"Look, Cheryl: I've jotted down three additional chapters from my book that I'd like you to pick up at the front desk. There's one on low-density foods, and in keeping with that, a chapter on how to like vegetables, and the one on learning to cook. They'll give you the info you need to move up to Step 6, which is refining your meals to goal size. Once you read those chapters, you'll be able to create quite a variety of meals within that 350-calorie range. Read them when you have time.

"I'd like to see you again in another two months. Have your blood drawn about a week before your appointment so we can review the results. This time, we'll not only check your sugar, but we'll recheck your cholesterol."

"Actually, I'd be really interested in seeing what my cholesterol is doing," Cheryl said. "I've certainly been eating much better than I used to." She took the slip Dr. Lang handed her.

"And Cheryl"—Dr. Lang looked up—"keep up the really good work you're doing. I know that learning to cook can be difficult, and maybe you think I'm asking too much, but just remember to take it one step at a time, just like you've been doing up to now. I truly believe you won't regret it."

"Thank you, Dr. Lang."

On the way home, Cheryl thought about learning to cook. She hardly knew how to throw a sandwich together, so how was she going to learn how to cook? *Well*, she thought, *two months ago, I couldn't salsa, and now I really look like I know what I'm doing.*

Cheryl read the chapter on low-density foods on the way home.

**What did Cheryl learn about creating
a satisfying 350-calorie meal?**

STEP 6: (PART 1) REFINING YOUR MEALS TO GOAL SIZE: THE LOW DENSITY METHOD
By
Nikki Lang, MD

Because this is meant to be a how-to book and not a complex justification of the information contained within, I have not and will not discuss at length the science of nutrition or dieting, except to give you as much information as you need to help you understand why certain things should be done. In the Appendix, you'll find some of the more complex information, if you so desire, but you do not have to read it in order to reach your goals.

Up until now, we have only talked about calorie limits in each of our meals, without limiting any of the meals by content. The reason I have emphasized the five smaller meals, and not stressed the calorie count as much, is that it is not always easy to create a satisfying meal in only 350-450 calories, which I am sure you have found out. There are probably that many calories in one slice of a large pizza, and I don't know of many people who would be satisfied at dinner with only one slice of pizza. So, how can we make meals that are tasty and satisfying, yet low in calories?

Studies have shown that satiety (feeling as if you've had enough to eat) is not judged by the amount of calories, but by the volume of food consumed—the actual amount of space that it takes up in your stomach. So foods that have a large amount of calories in smaller portions will not be as satisfying as foods that have fewer calories in a larger volume.

So what makes a food low-density? The more fiber and water contained within a particular food, the lower the caloric density, because water has no calories, and fiber is hardly absorbed by the body. Picking foods that are higher in fiber and water content allows us to eat far greater volumes of food with significantly fewer calories. What foods are we talking about? I'm sure you've already guessed, from the examples above, that this category is filled with mostly vegetables and many fruits. Adding many more of these foods to your diet repertoire will allow you to create far more satisfying low-calorie meals.

So understanding this concept, you can begin to realize the importance of vegetables and high-fibered grains in the diet: they allow you to eat more volume with fewer calories.

Let's look at an example of two meals, one high density and one low. A large DiGiorno pizza with pepperoni is 390 calories per individual slice, which would represent an entire meal. Or we could go with a KFC chicken breast that is 400 calories by itself. But neither option would be entirely satisfying as a meal. Now, suppose we chose instead to have a cup of vegetable soup (sixty calories); stacked eggplant made with spinach, feta cheese, roasted garlic, and marinara sauce* (158 calories); grilled or baked portobello mushrooms brushed with olive oil and garlic (75 calories); and a half cup of pasta shells (75 calories). By the time you finished this meal, you would be far more satisfied, and yet the calorie count of 368 is actually less than the one slice of pizza or the KFC chicken breast.

Another choice would be to eat half the chicken breast, a salad with low-cal dressing, and an ear of corn. Reducing the portion of high-density chicken leaves room to add a number of lower density foods, which allows for a more satisfying meal.

Low-density foods allow for larger meals and fewer calories.

If you've been following my instructions and are actually looking up the calories of the foods you eat, I'm sure you have found that vegetables and fruits, as a whole, have far fewer calories per volume than most other foods. I realize, of course, that perhaps you don't like many vegetables or fruits. This then brings us back to where we started. You must learn to acquire a taste for more and more vegetables to make this process work consistently.

---

*   Recipe taken from *Cooking Light Annual Recipes,* 1998

I talked about the methodology of learning to like diet drinks. In another chapter, we will discuss how these same principles can be applied to other foods, then I will make a variety of suggestions to again fool your palate.

As I mentioned earlier, the most important aspect of this process is making the concept of acquired taste work for you. The more low-density foods that you can learn to like and desire, the easier and easier it will become to find healthy and satisfying meals. It's not going to happen overnight, and you must want to make it happen. It's not impossible to lose weight without vegetables, high-grain breads, and fruits; Atkins has proven that. But to maintain a normal weight and enjoy your meals without ever dieting, more variety and balance is required so that you can chuck discipline and enjoy your life.

We have a lofty goal here. We are trying to create a change in habits that not only allows you to lose the weight, but keep it off "without really trying." It's not that it's really hard work. It's just that it requires perseverance and patience, which many of us have in short supply in this day and age.

Let's review our steps.

Step 1: **Stop drinking your calories**
Step 2: **Eat breakfast**
Step 3: **Eat a small meal between breakfast and lunch**
Step 4: **Eat an appetizer a few hours before dinner**
Step 5: **Find exercise that you enjoy.**
Step 6: **(Part 1) Refine you meals to goal size through the low density method.**

Chapter Thirteen

August 2005

"Mom, were you ever a good cook?" Cheryl asked that evening over dinner.

"I was, actually," Charlotte answered. "Before your father died, I used to enjoy cooking, but after his death, I just lost interest. It was too much trouble, and then by the time I might have regained interest, my health prevented me. Why do you ask?"

"Well, the doctor suggested today that I should learn how to cook, saying it would help me with healthy eating ... but you know, Mom, I don't even know where to begin. I thought that maybe if you knew how to cook, you could help me."

"I don't know, Cheryl. It's been so long since I've done any cooking. Why do you ask?"

"Dr. Lang gave me a chapter from her book on cooking. If I read it to you, maybe we could brainstorm and come up with some ideas. What do you think?"

"Sounds like a good idea." Charlotte smiled. "Heck, what else do we have to do?"

So, instead of running into her room to practice her dancing immediately after dinner, Cheryl read the entire chapter to her mom. She even ended up reading her the other chapter on low-density foods.

When Cheryl finished reading, Charlotte suggested that perhaps the first step she should take would be to buy some bags of frozen vegetables and experiment with them. And even if she liked the vegetables that came with the Lean Cuisines, she could eat the ones she cooked as well, adding bulk to her meal without a lot more calories. Cheryl thought this was a brilliant idea. She thanked her mom for her help before disappearing into her bedroom for her nightly practice session.

Cheryl was getting pretty good at salsa and felt ready to try one of the weekly parties at the dance studio. She thought she'd give Teresa a call and see if she would be free of the Italian stallion that night. The phone rang only once before Teresa picked up. "Oh, it's you," she said. "I was hoping it was Michael. We had a fight."

"What about?"

"Oh, something really stupid … not even worth talking about."

"Oh, c'mon, you know you want to talk about it," Cheryl coaxed. She knew her friend all too well. "Tell me anyway, even if it was stupid."

"Well, we were making plans to go out on Wednesday night, and I made a snide remark that maybe he could pick me up on time for once. It was really just a joke, but he got mad and told me that if I couldn't deal with his schedule, he didn't need to pick me up at all. Then he just hung up and hasn't called me back. That was two hours ago, and I don't really think I should call him back."

"Do you know why he's always so late?" Cheryl asked.

"A lot of it has to do with practice, and that he can't always get out on time. But if he knows that, why doesn't he just tell me a later time? Or why doesn't he just call when he realizes he'll be late? Sometimes he keeps me waiting for a couple of hours."

"A couple of *hours*? I agree," Cheryl commiserated. "It seems to me he should have more respect for your time."

"He respects me—"

Cheryl interrupted. "I didn't mean to say that he didn't respect you, I just meant that your time is valuable too. You work hard managing that store, and when you make free time to see him, he shouldn't keep you waiting like that. It's just not a considerate thing to do."

The other end of the line was silent.

"But, changing the subject entirely," Cheryl continued, not wanting her friend to get angry with her, "how about tomorrow we go to the open house dance party? I think I'm ready."

"Sure," Teresa said, "whatever."

"Good. It doesn't start until nine fifteen, so I can come home first and fix Mom dinner, then get changed. I'll drive, so I can pick you up."

Teresa agreed, but before Cheryl could say good-bye, Teresa exclaimed, "That's call waiting … gotta go! It might be Michael!" Just like that, she was gone.

Cheryl was happy despite the dial tone buzzing from the phone. She might get to see Victor tomorrow night. Maybe she'd wear a skirt. She looked a lot thinner in a skirt than she did in the hospital scrubs she usually wore.

*　　　　*　　　　*

When Teresa climbed into Cheryl's car to go to the dance studio, she was bursting with excitement. Michael had called her back and apologized. She told Cheryl how amazed she was. Although Teresa wasn't really sure he'd keep his promises to be more punctual, she was still very pleased that she had held her ground and not called him right back. Cheryl agreed that Teresa had done the right thing.

Initially, the dance party was a real dud. Cheryl realized she didn't know anyone, because she and Teresa were still taking private lessons. Maybe it was time to take group lessons … but then she wouldn't get a chance to see Victor that much. She wasn't sure he would even be here tonight, though she kept a hopeful eye out for him.

Teresa was asked to dance several times, and she actually did okay. That made Cheryl smile, because earlier Teresa had been more nervous than Cheryl—fretting about her dancing abilities. Cheryl was really happy for her, but no one asked Cheryl herself to dance. Then she spotted Victor. When he saw her standing alone, he came right over. Her heart skipped two beats.

"Hi," he said, "would you like to dance?"

Oh God, yes, she thought. *Thank you, thank you, thank you, Lord.* What she actually said was absolutely nothing—tongue-tied again. But, she did manage to nod.

He led her onto the dance floor, and they danced wonderfully. Her hours of practice were paying off; she could see it both in Victor's eyes and in the eyes of the crowd around her. Those eyes were looking at her, not with disdain, but respect. *They don't see a fat girl*, she thought in amazement. *They see a girl who can dance.*

When the dance was over, Victor thanked her for the dance and went to dance with another student. Cheryl thought that she probably wouldn't get to dance again the entire night … but she was wrong. Endless partners suddenly materialized, and some asked her to dance more than once. They were there to dance, and her performance had convinced them that she was the partner to have.

Both Cheryl and Teresa were absolutely exhausted by the end of the evening, but very happy. On the way home in the car, they discussed taking group lessons. But of course, Cheryl had one concern: would she get to see Victor?

"Maybe we should check the schedules," Teresa said. "I'll bet Victor teaches one of the group salsa lessons."

"Great idea," Cheryl responded. "Why don't you ask him when we take our lesson on Friday?"

"Fine by me," Teresa responded with a sly grin. "I know you're too shy to do it yourself!"

Cheryl grinned back, but all she would say as she dropped Teresa off at home was, "See you on Friday!"

When she flounced through her door, Cheryl really was on a high. She was hoping her mother would be up when she got home to share the excitement, but Charlotte was in bed, fast asleep.

The next day at lunch, Cheryl continued to brim with excitement over the previous night's events. "Tina," Cheryl said, "I know you guys have been teasing me about my gym bag, wondering what I've been up to. Do you really want to know?"

"Are you kidding? We've been dying to know. I just said to Darlene a little while ago that if you didn't tell us soon, I was going to strangle it out of you."

"Well," Cheryl said, dragging out the suspense a little longer, "what if I told you I was taking dancing lessons?"

"Dancing lessons? Why all the big mystery for dancing lessons? And here we thought you were staying overnight with some mystery lover. What kind of lessons?"

Cheryl was ready to tell them about the dancing, but not about Victor ... and besides, there was really nothing to tell. Granted, she had a huge crush on him, but he really hadn't given her the time of day and probably never would.

"No, no lover," Cheryl retorted. "I've been taking salsa lessons."

"Oooh, I've always wanted to learn the salsa," Tina replied. "Is it hard? Where are you taking the lessons?"

"Down on Second Street, at the Society Hill Dance Studio. It's not really that hard, but I will say it's a great form of exercise. That's why I started doing it. I needed the exercise, and that doctor you sent me to suggested dancing lessons. What a great way to work out! I knew I could never go to a gym, because I hate it so much. But dancing is so much fun. I didn't want to tell you guys about it, because I was afraid I might be a great big flop, and I didn't want to be embarrassed."

"So you're really enjoying it?"

"Absolutely! I went to one of their dance parties last night, and I had a ball—no pun intended. Initially, it was a little boring, because no one asked me to dance, so I just watched everyone else, but then my instructor came in and danced with me. After that, I had all the dance partners I could handle. It was really, really great." Cheryl beamed.

"When do you take lessons? I've always wanted to learn salsa."

"Right now, we're taking them on Fridays. Teresa and I share a private lesson. We're thinking of taking a class, but we don't know yet when the next class begins for the salsa. We were going to ask on Friday. If you're really interested, I'll let you know."

"Please do—I know I sure could use the exercise. Oh, and Cheryl, I wanted to tell you that I've noticed the weight you've lost. You look good."

"Thanks, Tina. Without you, I'm not sure I'd be doing as well as I am. My latest gig is learning how to cook. If you have any great but simple cooking ideas for some healthy meals, let me know."

"Well, I actually do know one off the top of my head. Have you ever eaten spaghetti squash?"

"No, but Dr. Lang mentioned it in a chapter I read on cooking."

"Do you know how to make marinara sauce?"

"Also, no. I told you I really don't know how to cook."

"It's really very easy. All you do to cook the spaghetti squash is to put it in a pot of boiling water for about twenty minutes. You just keep cooking it until it pierces easily with a fork," explained Tina.

"That sounds simple enough." Cheryl figured she could probably manage boiling water.

"The marinara sauce isn't much more difficult. All you do is take a large pot. Put in some olive oil—just enough to moisten the bottom of the pan. Throw in some chopped garlic. You can find garlic already chopped in a jar at the supermarket. Then toss in some chunks of onion and mushrooms, and if you want some peppers—green, yellow, red, orange—it doesn't matter. If you don't like peppers, just leave them out. Then open a large can of diced tomatoes and put that in there, along with maybe a third of a jar of store-bought marinara. The seasonings are important with marinara. Put in about a half of a teaspoon of oregano, a bunch of parsley flakes, about a half a teaspoon of pepper (more if you really like it spicy), a teaspoon or two of basil, a couple of bay leaves, salt, and maybe a teaspoon or two of sugar or Splenda. Let it simmer while your squash is cooking. Think you can do that?"

"That doesn't sound too complicated," Cheryl said hesitantly. "But maybe you could write it down for me? Also, I'm not clear on what you're supposed to do with the squash after it's cooked."

"Oh, sorry, that's the best part. You take it out of the pot and let it cool down some, and then you cut it in half. It remains too hot to handle for a while, so you'll want to use oven gloves. Once you clean out the seeds and stringy stuff, just like you would with a pumpkin or a cantaloupe, you then scrape out the shell, and the squash comes out in strands, just like spaghetti—hence the name spaghetti squash. Then you just plate the squash and put the marinara on top."

"I'd be willing to try it. Would you please write everything down so I can buy what I need at the supermarket tomorrow? Thanks."

Cheryl was going to give cooking a try. She just hoped that it worked out as well as the dancing had.

Change is difficult.
Learning to cook requires change.
Are you up to the challenge?

THE BENEFITS OF COOKING
By
Nikki Lang, MD

Throughout this book, many things I have said have made the assumption that you know how to cook. I realize, however, that many of you do not know how to cook. Perhaps your spouse or significant other does it for you. Perhaps you simply order out all the time, whether you're single or in a relationship. I have found that people who don't cook often have the hardest time controlling their weight. So, recognizing that fact, I would like to address this issue and suggest yet another new habit.

I am not suggesting that you become a gourmet chef. But the more you understand about cooking, as well as food in general, the greater your possibility of success in losing weight.

Another aspect of learning to cook is that it helps you appreciate the food you eat. Many people have the misconception that the cooks and the chefs of this world are always eating and are overweight. I won't deny that some chefs could stand to lose a few pounds, but the majority of people who love to cook, who savor their food and take pleasure in every mouthful, are not those who are significantly overweight. Quite the contrary: those who don't cook and eat only to fill their stomachs are the ones who don't always stop to appreciate the subtleties and nuances of the flavors passing over their tongues.

Knowing what seasonings or spices or cooking methods go into a meal, along with discovering which flavors you prefer, will help you to appreciate and savor what you're eating. Why is that even important? Because quality becomes more important than quantity!

Let me give you an example. Suppose the very first time you ever tasted a particular food—let's say, a piece of fish—it was either significantly overcooked or had a seasoning on it that you couldn't stand. Your response might be, "Yeccchhh, fish is terrible. I'll never eat fish again." Not understanding that the fish was overcooked, or not knowing the seasonings were actually the offending ingredients, tainted your view of fish in general, severely limiting your future diet repertoire. With experience in cooking, you would understand that the fish itself wasn't the culprit.

With regard to the quantity versus quality issue, let me give yet a different example. Most American meals are composed of a protein, a vegetable, and a starch. Why the starch? Rice, potatoes, pasta, and bread are generally bland foods with very little flavor. We all grew up with them, though; they're familiar and comforting. In truth, they are nothing more than fillers. When you're eating most of your calories in one or two meals a day, starches are needed to provide enough volume to the meal. But when you eat smaller meals, you will demand more flavor and less fillers. Why waste your calories on blandness? (I know—you really, really like them, but that's because they're a long-standing habit.)

So let's get on with it and figure out how to get you cooking a bit, if you don't cook already.

What makes a good cook? As with any skill, knowledge and practice play a huge role. The more knowledge and experience you have, the better you will become. If you attempt a dish you have never prepared with little or no knowledge, the chances of success are slim. Having said all that, you need to start somewhere.

I'm considered a fairly decent cook, but I can tell you I have made my share of disasters. Don't be afraid to try things. With each attempt, you learn, and that additional knowledge can be applied to your next venture.

If you can read, you can cook. Most recipes are self-explanatory, although some terminology or measurements might confuse you in the beginning. Make sure your first recipe is fairly simple and that you understand all of it.

Most of the mistakes that novice cooks make fall into two general categories: overcooking and poor timing. Food that is cooked too long is often dried out, tough, or stringy— or, if cooked in water, soggy or sticky. So you need to make sure that you follow the instructions precisely with regard to cooking time. You may want to cook something a shorter time than instructed, but test it to make certain it is done by either tasting it or cutting into it.

Overcooking often comes not from poor planning, but from distractions. How many times have we heard jokes or seen comedy routines about burned toast or roasts being charred in the oven? Getting distracted in this day and age is easy. A timer with a loud bell or buzzer can be very helpful with this problem.

Overcooking can also occur from a lack of knowledge or experience. Often, we eat foods a certain way because that's the way our parents did it, and it's what we're used to. One time, I was having dinner next to a pharmaceutical representative, and he ordered his steak well done. I couldn't help getting into a conversation with him about it. After all, steak cooked until it is well done tastes like shoe leather to me. We talked about it for some length, and he admitted that that was the way he had always eaten it. After some coaxing—he was a bit squeamish—I managed to get him to taste a piece of my steak, which had been cooked much less. By his own admission, it tasted better. On subsequent encounters, he informed me that he now eats his meat medium rare and enjoys it so much more.

Often, we overcook foods because we're afraid of disease. This has been taken much too far. Salmonella is the most common disease encountered when eating chicken. It is, however, only on the surfaces. (If you are cooking the chicken whole, you need to consider the cavity a surface as well.) Cooking all the surfaces thoroughly will kill any stray bacteria. If bacteria have invaded the substance of a piece of meat, it will have a rotting smell and consistency. If you cook chicken until it is no longer pink, it is finished. If you cook it longer, it will be dried out. A sautéed, pounded breast (one that has been beaten with a mallet to make it thinner) only requires about five to seven minutes maximum—sometimes less. If you are unsure, make a small cut into the center and look. If it's not pink, it's finished.

Pork, on the other hand, is finished cooking while it's still pink in the middle. Trichinosis, the parasite that invades pork, is generally not found in U.S. meats, but even if it is there, it will die at 137 degrees Fahrenheit. I usually cook my pork roasts to about 145 degrees, and in each case, the roast is still pink in the middle—and quite juicy, I might add. Cooked in this fashion, it doesn't even have to have gravy on it to taste good.

Fish also should not be overcooked. For deliciously moist fish, stop cooking as soon as translucency is gone. If you're not squeamish, you can safely cook most fish to a medium-rare consistency. As a sushi devotee, one of my favorite dishes is salmon cooked "Pittsburgh rare." This method leaves the fish very tasty and moist.

I'm not suggesting that just because I like my food less cooked, everyone should eat it that way. What I am suggesting is that you might like foods that you didn't like previously, simply because they were always overcooked, either by you or by someone else. Needless to say, the degree to which you prefer to cook something is a matter of personal taste. As we have discussed before, people enjoy what they are familiar with. If you like soggy green beans, then by all means cook your beans until they are soggy. But if you rarely eat green beans because you don't like them, maybe it's because you've only eaten soggy ones in the past.

Often, overcooking is a result of the second most common mistake: poor timing. When you cook a meal, it is important that everything you make is done at the same time. Many people lack a good sense of timing, so it is important that you plan ahead. Many foods can sit for a while and then be reheated, but some foods need to be served the moment they are done. You want to make certain that foods requiring immediate serving are not started before all other foods on the menu are completed or almost completed.

For example, let's say you're making fish, broccoli au gratin (with melted cheese sauce), and a salad. Let's also say that the fish only needs twelve to fourteen minutes to bake. You can prepare the fish so that it's ready to go into the oven. You can preheat the oven, but you'll want to make certain that you have already made the cheese sauce, prepared the broccoli to be steamed (with the water underneath already boiling) or microwaved, mixed the salad dressing, and set out the salad fixings, before putting the fish in the oven.

While the fish is in the oven, you can steam or microwave the broccoli until it's done—usually about five to six minutes, depending on the quantity—and put together the salad. Add dressing to the salad and toss, then add cheese sauce to the broccoli, and your fish will be ready. The salad hasn't been sitting too long with the dressing on it, so it won't be soggy. The broccoli remains on the slightly crisp side and doesn't get mushy in the cheese sauce. And the fish is brilliantly done, served hot out of the oven, but not overcooked and not sitting too long.

Timing is so very important to a good meal. Now, if you're making stew, that's not an issue. But let's say you're reheating some leftover stew, and you want to serve a fresh green vegetable with it. Since you don't want to overcook the vegetable, make certain the stew is getting close to warmed up before cooking the vegetable. If you put them on the stove at the same time, the vegetable will be done while the stew is still cold.

What you can see from my brief explanations is that preplanning is very important to the final outcome of the meal.

Now, if you're not much of a cook and have a microwave, you've probably never used it for much more than reheating coffee, popping popcorn, or cooking a prepackaged microwaveable meal. Believe it or not, your microwave can be one of your best allies in learning how to cook and making less of a mess.

Many foods can be cooked in a microwave with great success. I previously mentioned cooking broccoli in the microwave. Most vegetables (previously frozen) can taste even better that way. Because frozen vegetables were parboiled (very briefly placed in boiling water) straight from the fields before being frozen, they're not only amenable to microwave preparation, but they're often better than their unfrozen counterparts that have been sitting on the grocer's shelves for days. I have had corn from a frozen package that tasted fresher than "fresh" cobs of corn obtained from the supermarket.

Cooking frozen vegetables in the microwave is incredibly simple. Ignore the package instructions, if they tell you to add water. It's not necessary, since they automatically come with enough water in the form of frost, and adding more causes them to lose many of their nutrients. Just place a handful or two in a microwaveable bowl and add your seasonings, butter, oil, and so on. Cook for about three minutes on high. Take it out, give it a toss if it's not yet cooked, then put it back in again for another one to two minutes. A taste test might help you determine when the vegetables are done.

Not yet ready to eat? Put it aside and let it cool down. When you're ready to eat, put it back in the microwave to reheat for only about thirty to sixty seconds. You get the picture; experiment until you get the knack. The beauty of cooking in the microwave is that you can cook and serve in the same dish and save time on cleanup.

Although fish, meat, and fowl can be defrosted in the microwave, they should rarely or ever be cooked in a microwave. Protein cooks better slowly, thereby retaining moisture. Also, too many microwaves cook meat unevenly. At any rate, it's not for the novice.

What else can you cook in the microwave? Potatoes cook very nicely in the microwave, though if you want a crispy skin, you need to cook them in the oven. But you can bake a potato in the microwave in five to seven minutes, depending on the size of the potato and how many potatoes you put in there at one time. Just check them every few minutes by poking them with a fork. They're done when the fork meets little or no resistance. Don't forget to turn them over and place the side that was facing out toward the inside for more even cooking.

Corn on the cob is great in the microwave. A couple of ears of corn only take two to three minutes. You must, however, leave the corn in its husks, keeping the steam inside. More than a couple ears will take a bit longer. After a couple of minutes, take an ear out (wearing oven gloves) and check it by tasting the corn at the tip. If it doesn't taste done to you, put it back for another minute. Be careful not to overcook it, because even the cob will get soggy and limp!

What about spaghetti squash? Most squashes cook well in the microwave. Just remember, if you're going to cook them whole, to poke some holes in them so they don't explode. And make sure you check them frequently for doneness. Many squashes can be cut in half and seasoned before cooking.

This chapter is by no means an extensive lesson in cooking. It is, I hope, an encouragement to those who don't cook to give it a try.

There is no great mystery to cooking. You just have to give it a try, let yourself make mistakes, and stick with it. I'd like to end this chapter with a personal story that illustrates how important knowledge is in the cooking process.

My husband and I had previously had dinner at a friend's house and had enjoyed the ravioli she had served—so much so, that we'd asked her where she had purchased it. She told us, and my husband bought several packages of ravioli and put them in the freezer to use at a later date. He decided that his daughter would like the ravioli, so he placed it in the microwave to fix it for dinner. His daughter was a real trouper, trying very hard to chew what seemed like leather. She didn't want to hurt his feelings. My husband had been unaware that previously uncooked ravioli needed to be boiled in water. Because these were fresh ravioli purchased at a specialty store, they didn't come with instructions. This is an easy mistake for a novice to make. But I can assure you, he never made that mistake again.

So don't be timid. You might even surprise yourself. Cooking is really not that difficult, and it will make healthier eating an easier goal to reach. My most successful patients cook or learn how. You can too!

Chapter Fourteen

October-November 2005

On Friday, Teresa did ask Victor which group lessons he taught. It turned out that he wasn't giving any group salsa lessons, but he did teach swing to a group on Tuesday evenings. Over dinner that evening, Cheryl and Teresa decided to sign up for group salsa lessons with Luis. Teresa was very happy with that, because she had been getting a little strapped for cash. She had continued to take the private lessons because she hadn't wanted to disappoint her friend.

Cheryl also signed up for the Tuesday swing class with Victor, with plans to stay for the party afterwards. Her life took on a new rhythm. Charlotte continued to encourage Cheryl to go out, which she did regularly on Tuesdays and Fridays. On Wednesdays, Cheryl did the grocery shopping and spent the evening separating, packaging, and storing everything for easy access during the week.

Cheryl's cooking came along slowly, but surely. She learned to prepare chicken breasts, for example. Her mom told her how to get them thin by pounding them with a mallet. So on Wednesday nights, she pounded away, cutting the chicken breasts into smaller portions, then bagging them separately for easy defrosting. She also pounded pork tenderloins, having learned to prepare those as well. She even got a special defrosting tray. She learned how to make a few easy, low-calorie sauces that really perked up both the pork and chicken—so much so that her mom had started eating a little more. Charlotte even looked as if she were gaining a little weight.

The dance parties became more social for Cheryl. She wasn't always around Victor, so she slowly transformed from a mute into her usual animated, witty self. The other dancers enjoyed her company, and she was often surrounded by several people when Victor arrived. They still had their usual one dance, but her tongue began to unglue itself from the roof of her mouth, and Victor even laughed occasionally at her jokes.

Because Cheryl's comfort level had improved, Teresa had begun begging off from some of the dance parties, so she could spend more time with Michael before the football season had begun in earnest. Cheryl was surprised to discover that she was now comfortable going alone.

Cheryl continued to improve her eating habits, little by little. She even started bringing several meals with her to work. Between the regular exercise and healthier eating, she was losing weight steadily, at a slightly faster rate than Dr. Lang had expected. At her last visit, Cheryl had lost thirteen whole pounds. She weighed 208! Dr. Lang had said that she didn't want to see her again for three months, giving her no additional challenges. She wanted Cheryl to continue taking her medication; working on her cooking and exercise; adding to her knowledge base; and generally continuing to focus on the five small meals a day, keeping them in caloric range.

Tina joined the salsa class and occasionally came to the parties. At lunch the day after one of the studio's dance parties, Tina brought up the subject of having a party and inviting Victor. Cheryl was actually planning to have a party very soon, but hadn't really planned on inviting Victor. She wanted to have a party for her close friends to celebrate her breaking the 200-pound barrier, but when Tina made the suggestion, she realized that it was also close to Christmas, so she could have a dual party. Of course, she would only share the weight loss part of the celebration with her close friends, but wouldn't it be great for her mother to meet all of her new friends and see her dance as well? Perhaps she could get some help with moving the furniture in the living room and pulling up the rug to make it a real dance party. Cheryl's enthusiasm began to grow. Yes, of course, she would invite Victor. It would be only natural if she were going to invite others from the dance studio.

"You know, I think you have a really great idea, Tina. Do you think that you guys—I mean, you, Darlene, and Janie—could help me put the party together? I haven't entertained in eons, and I know I'm going to need some help."

"I know I'd love to help, and I'm sure they would too. Let's ask them."

Both Janie and Darlene were very enthusiastic and began offering suggestions right away, discussing what food, decorations, and the guest list. With a knowing smile, Tina inquired, "You are inviting Victor, aren't you?"

Cheryl blushed.

"You've been keeping secrets from us, Cheryl. Why don't we know about Victor?" Janie asked in a scolding voice.

"Because there's absolutely nothing to know. That's why!" Cheryl retorted. "Victor hardly knows I exist."

"Not true," interrupted Tina. "You don't see the way he gazes at you when you're not looking."

"You're just seeing things that aren't there," Cheryl responded adamantly. "I may be interested in him, but I know he's not interested in me. If he were, he would've done something about it."

"So says you. If you like him so much, why don't you do something about it?"

"I am. I am inviting him to my party. So there!" Cheryl walked out of the room to avoid further discussion. Dr. Weiner needed her anyway.

During the rest of the day, Cheryl pondered what Tina had said. *Does Victor really look at me that way? Is he really interested?* Cheryl couldn't imagine how someone so cute and suave could be interested in her.

Cheryl became consumed by her upcoming party. She had four weeks to plan it, and there was just so much to do. She set the date for the first Saturday in December and sent out invitations early so that most people would be free to come.

Planning the menu was even more difficult. There really wasn't enough time to talk about the menu at work. So she called Teresa, Wendy, Susan, and Carol to see if they could all get together and arrange a menu. She wanted everyone to enjoy the food, but she wanted it to be healthy food. That would require further brainstorming. She had plenty of ideas from the office staff but she wanted to get her friends' input. They agreed to meet on Sunday afternoon at three, but only if Teresa could have the football game on.

Sunday found the women around Cheryl's dining-room table with the Eagles game running in the background from the living room. Charlotte joined them. Cheryl had plenty of diet drinks available and some unbuttered popcorn for snacking.

"Okay," Teresa started, "Let's talk about drinks. I think there has to be beer and wine at a Christmas party, even though you guys don't drink that much. What do you think, Cheryl?"

"Oh, sure, but I haven't a clue how much to get. Do you?"

Susan asked, "How many people do you expect? Any idea?"

"I'm hoping about thirty-three," Cheryl answered.

"That many?" her mother asked, surprised her daughter had that many friends she didn't know about.

"Yeah, Mom."

Susan continued, "Well, I think we can we figure about half a bottle of wine for each. Some, of course, will drink more and some less, so I guess in the wine department, you should get about nine bottles. Make that ten—five red and five white. Leftover bottles won't spoil."

"Good." Cheryl continued, "So how much beer do we want, and shouldn't it be low-cal?"

"I would suggest a case of light beer, like Coors or Bud Light, and a case of Dock Street—that local beer I told you about," Susan said. "I know it sounds like a lot, but as I said before, it won't go bad."

Cheryl actually didn't mind having the leftovers. She knew from the dance parties that Victor liked both wine and beer. Maybe, just maybe, it would come to good use.

Teresa was only half listening, since most of her attention was on the game. Cheryl said, "I thought I'd get plenty of soda—mostly diet. But for those who can't stomach diet, I'll get a few regular ones. That too won't go to waste, so I'll just stock up. Drinks are the easy part. The hard part's going to be the food. I don't want to serve junk!"

Wendy suggested, "A vegetable platter with various dips is always good. You can buy the veggies already cut up as well and get premade, healthy dips. Whole Foods has a wonderful selection."

"That sounds like a great start," Cheryl continued, "but what else can we serve? I'd like to have some real dinner food so that people don't have to go anywhere else. I want them to stay and dance."

"My heavens, Cheryl!" her mom exclaimed. "Where are we going to have room for dancing?"

"Oh, I forgot to tell you, Mom. I've recruited some of my friends to help move the furniture in the living room to make a dance floor. We'll take up the rug, and I'll move my stereo in from the bedroom for the music. I've been collecting some CDs for that purpose. I'm going to see if I can get one of my acquaintances from the studio to burn a nice mix of dance music."

"So, back to the menu," Wendy interjected. "What about a chicken dish made with red peppers, snow peas, shiitake mushrooms, and mushroom sauce?"

"Mmmm, that sounds delish. Are you offering to make it for the party?"

"I will if you want me to."

"Sold!" said Cheryl. "Anyone offering anything else?"

Teresa finally took part. "I can make a mean vegetable lasagna with mostly low and nonfat cheese, and it's still really good."

"This is getting better and better. Thanks, Teresa. What if I make several kinds of salads with different dressings available?"

Susan hadn't yet offered anything other than advice, so she volunteered as well. "What do you think about bruschetta made on thin, toasted pita bread triangles as an appetizer?"

"What a great idea!" Teresa agreed.

"What's bruschetta?" Cheryl asked.

"It's basically diced tomatoes made with olive oil, garlic, and fresh basil."

"That sounds really good and healthy!" Cheryl was delighted. "Do you think maybe we should have one more dish to make sure we don't run out of food?"

"Probably," both Wendy and Susan said simultaneously. "But what?" Wendy added.

Everyone fell into thoughtful silence, searching their minds for a relatively simple, healthy dish.

"How about a roasted pork loin?" Carol finally suggested. "If you trim all the fat off, it's actually rather healthy. That's why they call pork the 'other white meat.' It's much leaner than beef, and cooked to the right temperature, it's safe and still moist."

"I just bought a meat thermometer—I could do that," Cheryl said excitedly. She wanted to contribute more to her own party, but she didn't want to try anything too difficult. The roast was just the ticket.

With most of the menu settled, the conversation turned to another subject, one particularly near and dear to most women's hearts: shopping.

Cheryl was ready to buy some new clothes. Most everything she had was much too big on her. She spent most of her present life in scrubs and sweat suits, so she was reluctant to spend a lot of money on stuff that, hopefully, she wouldn't be able to wear in another six months. She did, however, want to get something special for the party—something that Victor would notice.

The women arranged a group shopping spree. Her friends wanted to help her find just the right outfit. They too wanted Victor to notice her.

By the time Cheryl crawled into bed that night, she was both exhausted and stimulated. It had been a long day, but an exciting one. She was thrilled about the party and the menu. She was so happy that the girls had agreed to help her find the right outfit. It was exciting to contemplate Victor finally noticing her. She tried to sleep, but she couldn't. While lying restlessly in the dark, she suddenly remembered the two chapters that Dr. Lang had given her that she hadn't yet gotten around to reading.

Cheryl turned on the bedside lamp and looked around her room. She couldn't remember where she'd left those chapters. Her eyes fell upon the *Glamour* magazine lying on her night table. Some sheets of paper stuck out from underneath. Yup, these were the ones she was looking for. She grabbed them and crawled back into bed. She figured that reading about measurements and labels was bound to put her to sleep.

And she was so right. By the time she'd finished the chapter about measurements, she could hardly keep her eyes open. She'd save the chapter on nutritional labels for another night. She turned off her lamp and promptly fell asleep.

What did Cheryl learn about weights and measures?

UNDERSTANDING MEASUREMENT
By
Nikki Lang, MD

While examining the foods that you're eating, you may find four confusing measurement issues:

1. Calories are calculated in grams, which is a weight measurement.
2. Grams are a metric weight measurement, and in this country, we use pounds and ounces.
3. Ounces can be both a weight measurement and a volume measurement, and there is no relationship between the two.
4. Servings are frequently listed by volume, even though the caloric information is by weight.

So how can we make measurements less confusing and easier to understand so that you can gauge your portions and caloric intake accurately? Bureaucrats have threatened to switch the United States to the metric system for many years, but this change doesn't seem imminent. Oddly enough, we inherited the pound and ounce system from the British, and yet they went metric more than ten years ago and we're still stuck with their medieval system.

The metric system is much easier than ours, because it uses simple multiples of ten. So 100 grams is a centigram, and 1/1,000 of a gram is a milligram. (Most medications are listed in milligrams.) Also, 1,000 grams is equal to a kilogram. You don't have to divide by any odd numbers like we do when measuring something less than a pound.

The problem, of course, is that since you didn't grow up with these measurements, it's hard to comprehend what they translate into. We know what a pound of butter represents, and it's easy to picture how much that is in our heads, but what does a kilogram of butter look like? We have some idea what the size a McDonalds quarter pound patty looks like, but have no idea what part of a kilogram it is. Here is a table of equivalents to help you out.

1 kilogram = 2.2 pounds
500 grams (.5 kilograms) = 1 pound and 1.5 ounces
(essentially 1 pound)
28.35 grams = 1 ounce (this can be rounded to 30
for convenience)
100 grams = 3.5 ounces

So you can see from this table that a quarter-pound (4 oz.) hamburger weighs a little bit more than 100 grams, just like a quarter pound of butter. If something weighs just over 100 grams, you can get a sense of how much that represents by picturing those two items.

Now, calories are listed in single grams. Here's a table of equivalents.

1 gram of carbohydrate = 4 calories
1 gram of protein = 4 calories
1 gram of fat = 9 calories

If our quarter pound hamburger was *pure* protein without any fat whatsoever, it would have over 400 calories (4 x 100 grams). A quarter pound of butter, if it were pure fat, would contain over 900 calories. If you check out the paper wrapping on a stick of butter, the markings will show you how much a tablespoon of butter is and tell you that there are eight of these in the stick.

If you look up oil or butter in a calorie-counting book, you'll find that each tablespoon contains approximately 100 calories. If you multiply each tablespoon by 100 calories, you would get only 800 calories, not over 900 as I stated above. That is why I emphasized the word "pure." Foods are never pure carbohydrate, fat, or protein. There are always other substances mixed in there.

Take our hamburger, for example. It isn't just protein. It also contains fat and water and perhaps even a trace of carbohydrates, depending on how it's made. We will discuss this further in the chapter on nutritional panels. Just remember that foods are never purely carbohydrate, fat, or protein. They also may contain water and various types of fiber.

Let's now examine the issue of ounces. Both pounds and cups have ounces. Unfortunately, although the volume ounce and the weight ounce are similarly named, they bear no relationship to each other. Take flour, for example. A cup of flour would have 8 volume ounces, while it actually only weighs 4.75 ounces. Most vegetable servings are approximately 3 ounces by weight, but can vary in volume from 1 1/4 cups (broccoli, 10 volume ounces) to as little as 3/4 of a cup (peas and green beans, 6 volume ounces).

Remember when we discussed low-density foods and the importance of volume to appetite satisfaction? This discrepancy between volume and weight plays a large role in that concept. Be very careful when studying food content. Don't confuse liquid or volume ounces with weight ounces.

Lastly, although our serving sizes are frequently given in volume measurements, the calories are always expressed in weight. Fortunately, you can always find the weight measurement in grams in parentheses after the volume measurement.

Hopefully, you will no longer feel confused by weights and measurements. You don't have to be good at math to figure this stuff out; you just need to be careful not to mistake an apple for an orange (metaphorically speaking, of course).

Chapter Fifteen

December 2005

Cheryl had spent the entire week putting up Christmas decorations for her party. She wanted the place to look really festive. She went to Home Depot, bought several hundred extra lights, and tacked them up all over the living room and dining room. She even hauled out the fake Christmas tree from the basement and chuckled to herself when her first thought was, "Hey, this is good exercise!" She would've liked to have had a real one, but with all the other preparations, she decided it would be too much additional work. She did, however, decorate with fresh pine roping, and the scent permeated the house. The tree was set up in the entrance hall, welcoming guests with holiday cheer.

Cheryl looked around. The house was almost perfect; it was just missing the candles. Charlotte gushed, "Darling, it's absolutely beautiful. Why, with all the poinsettias, pine garlands, and lights it looks like a fairyland. I didn't know you were that creative, Cheryl." The truth be known, Wendy had helped some, but most of it had been Cheryl's idea.

Cheryl then insisted that Charlotte take a nap. She wanted her to save her energy for the party.

Her co-workers had come over earlier in the day and moved most of the furniture out of the living room before helping with some of the decorations. They put the furniture out in the garden with some tarps over it—despite the lack of snow in the forecast, no one was taking any chances. The beer and wine were on ice. Someone had to run out and get a wine opener, which Cheryl's kitchen was lacking.

Everything was almost ready, so Cheryl decided to shower and change. Wendy, Susan, Carol, and Teresa were coming early to bring food, but also to share in a small pre-celebration. Cheryl didn't want to lose sight of the original reason for the party. She indeed weighed less than two hundred pounds: 198, to be exact. She set two bottles of champagne on ice, one alcoholic and one nonalcoholic, to make the celebration complete.

As she got ready, Cheryl admired herself in the mirror. She had purchased a beautiful red dress at her friends' impish urging. It was a little more audacious than anything she was used to wearing. It was fairly low cut and fitted in the bodice, which showed off her large but still firm breasts. The waistline was also fitted (*I actually have a waistline now!*), and from the waist, the skirt flowed gracefully to mid-calf. The skirt was cut on the bias, so when Cheryl twirled, it lifted into an almost perfect circle. The dress was sleeveless, but it had come with a small bolero jacket that ended at the waist.

Cheryl twirled around in front of the mirror. She watched her skirt lift and show off her legs. She had nice legs, and they looked even nicer now that she had lost so much weight. She wore her hair pulled back, with strands hanging from the sides and a few wispy bangs. The hair stylist called it her "just got out of bed look."

For the first time in many, many years, Cheryl felt attractive. *Victor just can't help but notice me tonight,* she thought. She gazed at her reflection, grateful and proud that she was no longer the hopeless fat girl crying in a mall dressing room.

Cheryl went back out to the living room and started lighting candles. She put them all over the house wherever she could find a safe spot, then roused her mother to help her get dressed.

"Oh, darling," Charlotte exclaimed, "You look devastatingly beautiful tonight."

"You're prejudiced, Mom," retorted Cheryl, gratified nevertheless with her mother's remark.

"No, sweetheart, I mean it. You really are pretty. I don't think you have any idea."

"Mom, I know I've lost weight, but I'm still kind of fat."

"Ample, sweetheart, ample! Why, in Renoir's time, you'd be the absolutely perfect weight," Charlotte responded.

Cheryl helped her mom get dressed and helped her with some makeup, thoroughly pleased with her mother's comments. Cheryl then helped Charlotte into her now-decorated wheelchair. Cheryl was in red, her mother in green. They looked very Christmassy together.

Cheryl wheeled her mother out into the living room.

"Oh, Cheryl! The candles really are the final touch. You've done a magnificent job."

Cheryl went over to the CD player and put on some Christmas music. Just then, the bell rang, and the door opened. *Perfect timing.*

"We're here!" Wendy, Susan, Carol, and Teresa shouted in unison.

"Come in, and put your stuff down in the kitchen," Cheryl directed. "I'll call Mrs. Curtis so she can put some of the food in her oven. Oh, I'm using my room for coats, so you can put them in there."

Cheryl went into the kitchen to get glasses and both bottles of champagne. She handed the second bottle to Susan, and the two women each opened a bottle with a pleasant pop. She handed a glass to her mom and poured a generous amount into it. Everyone except Carol had the regular champagne.

Once all the glasses were full, Cheryl spoke up. "I want to propose a toast. This toast is to all of my close friends—and Mom, you're included in that group—without whom tonight would've never happened. With your support, I was able to get below two hundred pounds, and I know that I would never have gotten even this far if it hadn't been for you guys. Thank you."

Everyone took a sip of champagne. "Cheryl, you look really pretty tonight." Wendy was the first to say so, but Cheryl had caught a few admiring glances.

Susan added, "That dress was absolutely the right choice. If Victor doesn't notice you tonight, he's blind."

"And the house looks amazing," Teresa said, looking around at everything. "The lights and the candles are just stunning. It almost feels like I'm in a storybook—like *The Night Before Christmas* or something."

"Doesn't it?" Charlotte agreed vociferously.

It wasn't long before the other guests started arriving. The party became very lively very quickly. Over the next half hour, twenty people or so arrived, and Cheryl became busy playing hostess. She introduced everyone and made sure that all had drinks. The hors d'oeuvres were plentiful, and Susan's bruschetta was a big hit.

A short time later, Victor arrived, along with some others from the dance studio. When Cheryl introduced him to her mother, he bowed, took her hand, and kissed it. Cheryl could tell that her mother loved it. She clearly thought Victor was marvelous.

Since Victor was the only instructor there and Cheryl was the hostess, everyone agreed that it was only fitting that they begin the dancing. Cheryl was delighted by the suggestion. She found some swing music, and they were off. Cheryl danced with such expertise that it was becoming hard to figure out who was the instructor and who was the student. She was graceful and quick on her feet. When dancing, she moved with the ease of someone much lighter.

When the dance was over, Cheryl found the party-mix CD, which had some soft music mixed in with the swing and salsa music. She put that on, then asked one of the other students from the studio to dance, as did Victor. Soon it was hard to find enough space to squeeze onto the dance floor.

Cheryl glanced over at her mother and her bridge buddies from time to time. They were seated in a corner of the living room, where some of the chairs had been pushed aside, gabbing away animatedly while watching everything that was going on. Cheryl was pleased that they were smiling and laughing. It made her happy to see that her mother appeared to truly be enjoying herself.

Teresa kept telling Cheryl she should ask Victor to slow dance. Cheryl wanted to, but she was too nervous. *I just learned to* speak *to this guy ... as nervous as I am, I'm not sure I could even get the question out!* So she asked a number of the other students. After dancing with three or four others, Cheryl finally forced herself to ask Victor. *You've come this far. You can do this.*

The words were barely out of her mouth before Victor rewarded her with a warm smile and a nod. She was so happy in Victor's arms, she was radiant. When her mother caught her eye over Victor's shoulder and gave her a thumbs-up, Cheryl couldn't help but smile.

Eventually, Cheryl put the Christmas CD on and told everyone it was time to eat. Everything tasted superb. Cheryl's pork roast was perfect. For dessert, she had fresh fruit salad. She did serve vanilla ice cream for those not watching their weight and indulged herself with one heavenly dollop.

The rest of the night passed in a rapid blur of dancing, talking, and drinking. By the time everyone finally left, the tired hostess was ready to be alone. It had been a wonderful evening. She was very proud of herself. She had planned well, and it all had gone perfectly. *Well ... almost perfectly*, she retracted. Victor still hadn't asked her out. She began to wonder if that was ever going to happen. Her friends said otherwise, but what if Victor was just interested in her as a friend?

Cheryl took off her shoes. Her feet were sore from standing and dancing on them all night. Admittedly, she was tired, but not yet ready for bed. She walked around picking up dirty glasses and trash and generally tidying up a bit. She didn't want to face such a complete mess in the morning. She gradually worked her way into the bedroom. Before changing into her pajamas, she looked at herself in her beautiful new red dress. She was really starting to get a waistline again, and if she stared really hard in the mirror, she could just glimpse the beautiful woman that her mother had referred to earlier. That woman was there; she just needed to be unveiled.

As Cheryl got into bed, she spied the still unread chapter on nutritional labels. *No time like the present,* she thought. She read the chapter with great interest. She'd recently heard a doctor interviewed on TV who stated that everyone who was overweight knew what to do; they just had to make up their minds to do it. *How wrong could he be? I guess most doctors don't know a great deal about nutrition. I'm really lucky I met Dr. Lang.*

She put the chapter down and turned off the lights. As her eyelids drooped, she promised herself to read more nutritional labels from here on out.

Most people have problems accurately reading nutritional labels.

Learn what Cheryl learned, and you won't be most people.

DECIPHERING NUTRITIONAL LABELS
By
Nikki Lang, MD

Some parts of a nutritional label are very simple to understand, but manufacturers generally still manage to make labels more complicated than necessary. The labeling of some parts of the nutritional panel is absolutely diabolical.

I have often imagined that the bureaucrats responsible for label standards make them as complicated as they can so that few will understand; maybe it makes them feel smarter. Or perhaps they represent a secret club and want to keep the information to themselves. I'm joking, of course, but as we discuss some of the labeling issues later on in this chapter, you'll wonder about the wisdom of government labeling requirements.

Fortunately, the easy part of the labeling is the part we are most interested in. As we discussed in the previous chapter, manufacturers are required to specify the contents of any food package in both U.S. measurements and standard gram measurements. We know that the U.S. measure may be either a volume measurement or a weight measurement, while the standard gram measurement is always in weight, never volume.

When we look at food labels, we are most interested in how many calories there are in a serving, as well as how much of those calories come from fat, protein, and carbohydrates. If we're smart enough to have other health concerns aside from weight issues, we'll also want to know what types of fat and carbohydrates are included. I have copied the labels from two cereals, both marketed as "healthy" high-fiber cereals. Let's examine these labels together to help us understand the information—and hopefully begin to appreciate the importance of interpreting it properly.

Nutrition Facts
Serving Size 1¼ cups (55g)
Servings Per Container About 7

Amount Per Serving	Fiber One Honey Clusters	with ½ cup skim milk
Calories	170	210
Calories from Fat	10	10
	% Daily Value**	
Total Fat 1g*	**2%**	**2%**
Saturated Fat 0g	**0%**	**0%**
Trans Fat 0g		
Polyunsaturated Fat 0g		
Monounsaturated Fat 0g		
Cholesterol 0mg	**0%**	**1%**
Sodium 170mg	**7%**	**10%**
Potassium 120mg	**3%**	**9%**
Total Carbohydrate 47g	**16%**	**18%**
Dietary Fiber 14g	**59%**	**59%**
Soluble Fiber 3g		
Sugars 5g		
Other Carbohydrate 28g		
Protein 3g		
Vitamin A	0%	4%
Vitamin C	0%	0%
Calcium	10%	25%
Iron	25%	25%
Vitamin D	0%	10%
Thiamin	25%	30%
Riboflavin	25%	35%
Niacin	25%	25%
Vitamin B₆	25%	25%
Folic Acid	25%	25%
Vitamin B₁₂	25%	35%
Phosphorus	10%	20%
Magnesium	8%	10%
Zinc	25%	30%
Copper	2%	2%

* Amount in cereal. A serving of cereal plus skim milk provides 1g total fat, less than 5mg cholesterol, 230mg sodium, 330mg potassium, 53g total carbohydrate (10g sugars) and 8g protein.
** Percent Daily Values are based on a 2,000 calorie diet. Your daily values may be higher or lower depending on your calorie needs:

	Calories	2,000	2,500
Total Fat	Less than	65g	80g
Sat Fat	Less than	20g	25g
Cholesterol	Less than	300mg	300mg
Sodium	Less than	2,400mg	2,400mg
Potassium		3,500mg	3,500mg
Total Carbohydrate		300g	375g
Dietary Fiber		25g	30g

Nutrition Facts
Serving Size 1/2 cup (30g)
Servings Per Container about 11

Amount Per Serving	
Calories 90	Calories from Fat 10
	% Daily Value*
Total Fat 1g	**2%**
Saturated Fat 0g	**0%**
Trans Fat 0g	**0%**
Cholesterol 0mg	**0%**
Sodium 55mg	**2%**
Total Carbohydrate 23g	**8%**
Dietary Fiber 8g	**33%**
Sugars 5g	
Protein 3g	
Vitamin A 0%	• Vitamin C 0%
Calcium 2%	• Iron 6%

* Percent Daily Values are based on a 2,000 calorie diet. Your daily values may be higher or lower depending on your calorie needs:

	Calories:	2,000	2,500
Total Fat	Less than	65g	80g
Sat Fat	Less than	20g	25g
Cholesterol	Less than	300mg	300mg
Sodium	Less than	2,400mg	2,400mg
Total Carbohydrate		300g	375g
Dietary Fiber		25g	30g

Calories per gram:
Fat 9 • Carbohydrate 4 • Protein 4

When we look at any label, the first thing we head for is the calorie count. We usually don't even bother looking at what constitutes a serving. Depending on the food we're buying, we will usually then look to either the fat or carbohydrate content. Nobody seems to pay much attention to the protein. Unless you're a strict vegetarian, it doesn't seem to be an issue.

But if we take that approach with the labels above, we miss something important: the serving size. The cereal on the left not only markets itself as high fiber, but displays the amount of fiber that one serving contains in prominent writing on the front of the box. In very large letters, this cereal boasts over 50 percent of the 25-gram daily fiber requirement in just one serving. This makes it look really good in the fiber department. It certainly caught my eye, and I hurriedly assumed this cereal was going to give me the most fiber.

However, when I studied the label more carefully, I noticed the serving size on the "better" cereal: 1 1/4 cups. That's a large serving. When I took the time to measure how much cereal I would pour into a cereal bowl, I discovered that it's somewhere around 3/4 cup. So, in a realistic serving, I'm not actually getting 14 grams of fiber. In fact, I'm only getting a little more than 8 grams. But I'm also only getting 102 calories, not the 170 calories listed on the label. Not shabby, but let's look at the other label.

The label on the right lists 8 grams of fiber per serving, but it also lists a serving as only 1/2 cup. I already figured out that I eat about 3/4 cup of cereal for breakfast, so actually this cereal contains more fiber for the same serving size than the first one. Its packaging doesn't have any great big numbers on the front boasting the percentage of daily fiber it offers. However, if it upped its serving size to 3/4 cup, then it could claim 12 grams of fiber per serving, which is almost 50 percent of the daily recommended amount. If it upped its serving size to 1 cup (still less than the other cereal), the package could brag that one serving contains 16 grams of fiber—more than 60 percent of the daily fiber requirement. So, why don't they do that?

Well, let's look at the other factors.

The cereal on the right only advertises 90 calories per serving, but if it doubled its serving size to 1 cup, the calories would double as well. Many people would hesitate to pick up a cereal with 180 calories per serving without the milk. Also, that increase in serving size would bump the sugar content to 10 grams, which might make people shy away. But let's look at these two labels from a different aspect.

Both boxes of cereal were about the same size. I'm sure you've noticed that most cereal boxes are about the same size, with modest variations. However, one box contained only 12 ounces of cereal, while the other contained 15 ounces. Can you guess which one was the lighter box? If you look carefully at the labels, one box states it has 7 servings in a box, while the other one touts that it has 11 servings in a box. Now, have you figured it out? Right: the cereal that gives you only a 1/2 cup for a serving, the one with 11 servings, is the lightweight—the 12-ounce box. Isn't it really interesting how much thought, consideration, and marketing goes into a nutritional packaging label? It's usually reasonably accurate. In fact, I recently read a study that looked into the accuracy of nutritional labels and, for the most part, found them to be fairly precise. But isn't it fascinating how these labels, despite that accuracy, can be used to a manufacturer's advantage? By presenting the same facts differently, they show you what they want you to see. But you can be smarter than they are by actually learning to read these labels and making the right decisions.

Now, to be fair to the cereal company that had the 11 servings per package, I should mention that their cereal was far more dense. In other words, it weighed more per volume ounce. In fact, it weighed 2 grams more per volume ounce. So, you're getting more substantive food and less air for each volume ounce you eat. And, of course, we're paying for the food, not the air. On the other hand, aren't we more interested in less dense food so that it fills us up faster? If we do a few more calculations, we find that if the box contains 11 servings, and each serving is a 1/2 cup, then the entire box only contains 5 1/2 cups of cereal. The other box contained only 7 servings, but since each serving was 1 1/4 cups, its box contained 8 3/4 cups. Which box do you think you should buy?

My preference is for the box with only 7 servings. Although I'm not getting 14 grams of fiber per serving, I'm still getting 8 grams. Also, I'm taking in only 102 calories and still getting the larger 3/4 cup volume. And, in fact, the box actually contained over 11 servings, since I only eat 3/4 of a cup each time, and the other box only contained just over 7 servings of that size.

Before we continue examining these same two labels, let's just review what we've established so far.

When looking at a nutrition panel, it's very important to note the serving size before jumping down to the calorie count and other information. It's also important to note how many realistic servings are in a container. In the case of cereal, this consideration is not nearly as important as with other foods, since you aren't likely to consider an entire box a single portion. But nonetheless, from the information above, you can still see that serving size matters greatly, especially when comparing one cereal to another.

When looking at small containers, however—say, a can of tuna fish in water—it's very important to note that the tiny 6-ounce can has 2 1/2 servings. That way, when you pick up the can and quickly read "60 calories," you don't make the assumption that the entire can is 60 calories when the entire can actually contains 150 calories.

A small DiGiorno pizza, which appears to be a personal-size pizza, looks at first blush to be a single serving. At 300 calories, that doesn't seem like a bad deal, but upon closer inspection of the labeling, you'll find that this tiny little pizza supposedly contains three servings—making the entire pizza 900 calories! Egads, that's around half of an entire day's calories. Not a good choice.

Okay, we've discussed serving size and the calorie count, so let's move on to the nutrients. The first listing after calories is fat. The sublistings under fat are saturated fat, trans fat, polyunsaturated fat, and monounsaturated fat. Though cholesterol information is included on the label in the total fat calories, it doesn't appear as a sublisting.

As I mentioned previously with regard to weight loss, fat is fat is fat. The calorie counts are the same, regardless of what type of fat is contained within that particular food. However, if you want to eat healthily, or if you already have a problem with cholesterol, you want to keep cholesterol, trans fats, and saturated fats to a minimum. Recommendations are that you consume less than 300 milligrams of cholesterol per day and less than 20 grams of saturated fats. Ideally, you want to avoid "bad" fats as much as possible. Also, since fat has 9 calories per gram, whereas protein and carbohydrates only have 4 calories per gram, the less fat in a particular food, the more likely it is to be a lower-calorie food, although that's not guaranteed. Just because something is advertised as low fat does not automatically make it a healthy food, but it does increase the possibility of fewer calories. The important thing to remember is to keep fat content as low as possible and try to avoid saturated and trans fats.

Sodium (salt) and potassium are the next ingredients noted. These are only important if you have high blood pressure, problems with fluid retention, or other medical problems that may require either salt or potassium restriction. If you don't have any of these problems, sodium or potassium content is of little consequence.

However, I have met numerous young patients who avoid salt assiduously because they consider it unhealthy. They subsequently found out quite the opposite: salt is a very important part of our diet. All the salt in the world will not give someone high blood pressure. It's only a problem if you already have high blood pressure. Young active women who are otherwise healthy are doing themselves a disservice by restricting their salt intake. Some will even suffer syncopal episodes (loss of consciousness) due to insufficient salt intake, especially in hot weather, when their blood pressure drops too low. Salt is a very necessary ingredient to maintain a normal blood pressure. Yes, too little salt can be a problem, but for most people an average American diet has more than enough salt so this is rarely an issue.

The bottom line is if you have no medical reason to avoid salt, you can completely ignore this part of the panel. If you do have a problem with salt, you want to keep your intake below 2,400 milligrams (mg) per day.

The next category is carbohydrates. The subcategories of carbohydrates include: fiber, sugars, sugar alcohols, and other carbohydrates. With regard to weight loss, these subcategories are very important. Since fiber and sugar alcohols are only partially absorbed, they don't count significantly in the calculation of calorie content.

Nutritional panels include fiber and sugar alcohols in their total calorie count, but only partially, which makes it somewhat confusing.

Recently, I received a correspondence from Dreamfields, the makers of a relatively new low-carb pasta. I had asked them this question: if there are only five available carbs in each serving of their pasta, then why is the calorie count so high? Shouldn't the carb reduction have significantly reduced this number on their nutritional panel? The representative explained that this discrepancy had to do with government regulations, which the company is in the process of sorting out. Apparently our bodies absorb some minimal amount of the fiber contained within each serving, but it is significantly less than the 4 grams for standard carbohydrates. Also, I was led to understand from their literature that, although some portion of this fiber is metabolized and therefore counts as calories, it probably doesn't affect the glycemic index significantly, since the total absorption of these calories takes some time.

So, if you try to add up all the separately listed calories by nutritional categories, the sum can fall significantly short of the total calories included—or significantly over, if you don't subtract the fiber grams.

Let's look, for example, at one of the boxes of cereal.

If we look at the fat content, we see 1 gram of fat, which is equal to 9 calories. We see 47 grams of carbohydrates, but we are told that 14 of these grams are fiber (and therefore not absorbed like other carbs), so if we subtract the 14 from the 47, we get 33 net carbohydrates, which would be 132 calories (4 x 33). The last nutritional component, protein, is listed as 3 grams, which translates to 12 calories. So, the total calorie count would be 133 for carbohydrates, plus 9 for fat and 12 for protein, totaling 154 calories. The panel lists 170 calories in a serving. What happened to the other 16 calories? Each gram of fiber is counted as slightly over 1 calorie of absorbed energy. So, this accounts for the discrepancy, since the label lists 14 grams of fiber.

If we perform the same exercise on the other box of cereal, we come up with 60 calories from carbohydrates, plus 9 calories from fat and 12 calories from protein, totaling 81 calories. Again, we are short, slightly over the amount of grams of fiber in a serving.

The same holds true for sugar alcohols, which are also not fully absorbed like fiber, but are included in the total calorie count (at slightly over 1 calorie per gram). So, in the end, it all really does begin to make some sense. Again though, what is the bottom line? Believe the calorie counts that are given on the package, but do pay some attention to where those calories are coming from to make better decisions for you personally.

The next nutrient on a packaging label is protein. If you are not a strict vegetarian, this label information is not terribly important. Most American diets easily reach the 50-gram recommended daily intake. Four-ounce servings of most protein-rich foods (meat, fish, chicken) have approximately 30 grams of protein. Eggs have about 8 to 9 grams of protein, and a half can of tuna has about 20 grams. Even if you are a vegetarian, it is not difficult to achieve a 50-gram intake of protein. A cup of soybeans has about 18 grams of protein, and 3 ounces of tofu has over 11 grams of protein.

Believe it or not, we have finished discussing the *easier* portion of a nutritional panel. We are about to embark on the more mysterious aspects of these labels, which will make you wonder why on earth did government bureaucrats choose such a baffling manner of labeling?

If you examine the cereal labels under discussion, you will notice percentages following all nutrients. These percentages are derived from the daily recommended numbers for the intake of each of the nutrients listed. For fat, saturated fat, sodium, potassium, carbohydrates, and fiber, you'll find a listing at the bottom of each panel telling you what those numbers should be for a 2,000 and 2,500 calorie diet.

However, if you are on a 1,700-calorie diet, which I recommend for most women, you'd have to do an awful lot of figuring to glean your specific recommendations—and then try to adjust listed percentages accordingly. But in all honesty, why does it matter? Are we going to keep track throughout the day of the percentage of each nutrient we've already had? I don't think so. If we have a problem with a particular nutrient—let's say, sodium—then doesn't it make more sense to just keep track of the milligrams throughout the day so we know when we've reached our limit? What about cholesterol? To me, the only time it really makes sense to put down a percentage is when it is extremely high. Most people ignore these numbers anyway, because they make so little sense from a practical standpoint.

What we haven't discussed are the vitamins and minerals listed on the boxes. These are only listed in percentages. How silly is that? Does anyone know what the recommended daily allowance (RDA) is for any given food? Unlike with the other nutrients, milligrams of vitamins are not even listed on the package. Let's say you are particularly interested in your calcium intake. Any idea, by looking at a nutrition panel, how many milligrams of calcium you're getting? Not if you don't know what the recommended daily allowance is. Do they tell you anywhere on the box what the recommended amount is? On the one cereal panel, you are informed that, with 1/2 cup of milk, you're getting 10 percent of the vitamin D recommended for the day. Any idea how many milligrams that is? What if I told you that the recommended dose of vitamin D by most doctors is four times the RDA? Then the percentage listed on the side of the box should really be 2.5 percent. Shouldn't it?

I suppose labels don't list the actual milligrams or international units of these substances because the government feels that this data might confuse or intimidate the average person. Perhaps percentages are easier to understand, but without the baseline information, they are also absolutely useless.

If you really wanted to figure out how you could get the recommended daily allowance of calcium, you'd have to first find the information somewhere (not on any nutritional panel). Then, each time you looked at a panel, you'd have to figure out how many milligrams you were consuming by multiplying the percentage by the total requirement, then adding it all together.

I suppose some brilliant government employee figured out that you could just add up the percentages until you reached a hundred or greater. The problem with that system is that not every food we eat comes in a package with a nutritional panel. Suppose we eat some fresh foods as well? Then we can look up the amount of calcium in those foods, and it gives us the information in milligrams. How do we add that up with our percentages?

I think the whole percentage notion is truly a waste of time, and except at the extremes, should essentially be ignored … which I'm sure you've been doing anyway. At least, when I casually survey most people, they don't have a clue as to what those percentages mean. Putting this information on the panel, in the present format, I believe, is a mistake. It intimidates too many people into ignoring labels entirely.

Hopefully, you'll no longer be among the scores of people who totally ignore or misread nutrition facts and will begin to make label-reading a routine. It is prudent if you want to educate yourself and achieve a healthy diet.

P.S. A table in the Appendix lists the RDAs, if you're interested.

Chapter Sixteen

March 2006

Cheryl's visit to the doctor two weeks after her Christmas party was again successful. She weighed 196 pounds. Since Cheryl was making such good progress, Dr. Lang told her not to return for another three months. But when Cheryl returned in March, she had only lost seven pounds, and she wanted to know why.

"Dr. Lang, I'm still doing all the same things. I'm getting a lot of exercise with my dancing. I'm eating the five small meals a day. I'm not drinking any of my calories, and I hardly eat any junk food at all. What am I doing wrong?" Cheryl was frustrated. She thought she should have lost much more.

"Let's review your chart and see what we can come up with. When you originally came to see me in April of last year, you weighed 235 pounds. I told you then that you shouldn't expect a weight loss of more than three or four pounds per month. It's been eleven months, which means I would've expected you to lose thirty-three to forty-four pounds. Instead you've lost forty-six pounds. That's excellent, Cheryl! Now, the other thing you have to consider is the closer you get to your goal weight, the slower your weight loss is going to be."

"Why is that?"

"Because you weigh less, you actually burn fewer calories doing the same activity. For example, when you first started dancing, you weighed about forty pounds more than you do today. Imagine dancing now with forty pounds of weight strapped to your body. Do you think you would burn more calories?"

Cheryl was beginning to understand what Dr. Lang was getting at.

"You could, however, wear a weight vest during your practice sessions at home. That will help build muscle as well as burn a few extra calories."

"Why is building muscle important? I honestly think my muscles are big enough. I don't want bulging muscles."

"I'm sure you don't. Don't worry: lifting heavy weights is what gives people bulging muscles. Like we've discussed, what you want to do is increase the overall muscle mass in your body so that you naturally burn more calories, even when you're not doing anything.

"By wearing more weight while you practice your dancing, not only can you increase muscle mass, but you can also burn more calories, because you'll be working harder. If you can get other types of muscle-building exercises in during the day, that will help as well. Let me give you some that you can do while at work. I realize you don't like to do 'exercise' exercise, but maybe you can give it a try, since it'll help you lose weight faster."

Having provided Cheryl with a cursory review of the exercises, Dr. Lang proceeded with some other ideas. "I'd also like to discuss another way to lose weight a bit faster—but with caution."

Cheryl was interested in anything that could speed up the process.

"You've done the Atkins Diet, right?"

Cheryl nodded.

"Do you have any idea how or why it works?"

Cheryl shook her head.

"When you eat absolutely no carbohydrates, your insulin levels remain very low, and without a rise in insulin, all the food you've eaten cannot enter the cells and simply floats around in your bloodstream, unused, until the body discards it. It's the equivalent of fasting. Now, do you remember the inherent danger to fasting?"

"Slowing my metabolism?"

"Exactly right! And the last thing we want to do is slow up our metabolisms … so how can we put that information to good use?"

Cheryl shrugged.

"There are two ways. The creator of the South Beach Diet came up with one. If you eat just a little bit of carbohydrates along with your protein, you only absorb some of it."

"I think I understand. What's the other way?"

"You can do Atkins for just one or two days in a week. You should eat a regular small breakfast to jumpstart your metabolism, like you've been doing, and then do Atkins for the rest of the day. The next day, you should resume your original routine. If you do it for that short a time, your metabolism isn't in jeopardy, and you've essentially eaten 1,400 fewer calories for the day. You just have to be really careful not to overdo it. The last thing you want to do is slow your metabolism.

"Let me give you a chapter on the high-protein method I'm speaking of. You can pick it up at the front desk, along with a copy of the desk-side exercises I mentioned earlier. I want you to come back again in three months, but don't hesitate to come back sooner if you're confused or frustrated."

Dr. Lang stood up and reminded Cheryl, "Now don't forget to schedule an appointment in three months—sooner if you need to. Let's keep you on the right track."

Cheryl was in full agreement with that. She also felt a little better, now that quicker weight loss seemed possible. She would read the new chapter and see if she could come up with a plan. *There really is a lot to learn,* she thought.

Cheryl read the chapter on the bus ride home. She looked at the desk exercises as well, but doubted she would actually do any of those.

Know thyself, she thought wryly. *Isn't that what they say? Well, at least I'm finding solutions that work for me.*

Can understanding a low-carb diet relieve some of your frustration?

STEP 6: (PART 2) REFINE YOUR MEALS TO GOAL SIZE: THE HIGH-PROTEIN METHOD
By
Nikki Lang, MD

Before embarking on this discussion, let's review food-group basics to make sure we're on the same page. There are three separate groups of food: protein, fat, and carbohydrates. Without exception, all the food we eat falls into these three categories. Protein generally comes from living things—fish, fowl, and four-legged mammals (pigs, steer, sheep, and so on). Some plants, though, are also very high in protein, such as soybeans and most nuts.

Fat, too, comes primarily from living things, but it also can come from plants—though generally it needs to be extracted from large quantities of those plants. You know this intuitively, because you've purchased it at the supermarket: corn oil, safflower oil, and just plain vegetable oil. Nuts are a good source of oil as well; most of us are familiar with peanut oil, but you can purchase oil extracted from almost any other common nut.

Just about everything else that I haven't already mentioned is a carbohydrate. Needless to say, that covers quite a broad range of foods. All fruits and vegetables are carbohydrates. All grains are carbohydrates, as well as everything that one makes from grains, whether it's cereal, pasta, or baked goods. Sugar cane, a major source of sugar, is a carbohydrate. Almost everything that falls into the category of "junk food" is a carbohydrate. See why giving up carbs for the rest of your life is a bit unrealistic?

Now that you have a better understanding of the different categories of food, let's improve your understanding of the high-protein method.

Previously, we'd mentioned the Atkins Diet and stated that it allowed you to lose weight without eating fruits, vegetables, and high-fiber grain products. This might seem like the ideal diet for vegetable haters. The problem, however, is that it doesn't permit any carbohydrates (original Atkins, not the modified version) at all. That means no bread, bagels, rice, potatoes, baked goods of any kind, or even the occasional vegetable or piece of fruit. You're allowed to eat an unrestricted amount of calories, as long as all the calories come from protein or fat. That's right: you can eat all the steak you want, or you can have as many eggs or strips of bacon you want. You can even snack on pork rinds. If you're a meat eater and hate vegetables, it sounds great … but you can't eat any car-bohydrates at all. And who can do that for any length of time? You will lose a lot of weight very quickly, but can you stay on this diet forever? Remember the consequences of this type of diet. (If you've forgotten, it might be a good idea to reread chapters five and nine.)

You must be asking yourself, how can this possibly work? How can you eat all those fatty, densely caloric foods and lose weight? It just doesn't make any sense. Where does all that food go if you eat it and don't put on any weight? Good question!

The Atkins Diet is based on a brilliant concept, and Dr. Atkins held to its tenets despite the derision of the medical community for many years. He did ultimately modify his principles somewhat in the interests of a healthier diet, but maintained that his original diet was a healthy one.

Well, it is, and it isn't. The reason that Atkins works is that, without insulin, the body is unable to absorb and process any of the nutrients that are in the blood-stream. Sugar (glucose, more specifically) is what stimu-lates insulin levels to rise. If you eat nothing that can be converted quickly to glucose, the insulin levels will remain too low for your body to absorb most of the food you are eating. When you eat only protein and fat, your body remains in a state of catabolic metabolism (break-ing down). Your body will use ketones for energy instead of sugar. As a result of being on a strict protein diet (no carbohydrates whatsoever), you are putting your body through the equivalent of fasting, and what does that do to your metabolism? You guessed it: slows it down even more. So what happens when you go off the Atkins Diet? You know the answer.

Another issue to contend with, as an aside, is the health of the Atkins Diet. Eating all those bad fats has to be unhealthy, right? Shouldn't your cholesterol go sky high on this diet? Not really. If you stay on the diet and remain quite strict about it, your cholesterol will actually go down, because you're not absorbing these foods. But the consequences of cheating are severe; you could be doing a great deal of harm to both to your health and your diet. All those extra not-so-nice energy molecules are floating around in your system with no place to go. If you cheat and give your body some sugar, or anything that can be converted to sugar—within hours of consuming all this protein and fat—then you raise your insulin levels, and now your body will absorb all those nasty molecules with a vengeance.

So in reality, there is nothing wrong with the Atkins Diet, either from a weight-loss or health perspective. But human nature prevents the Atkins Diet from working; the diet is not practical for a prolonged period of time in our busy lives. Therefore, we will cheat and cheat again, and subsequently reject the diet entirely.

I have seen this over and over again with numerous patients. When I broach the subject of the diet's failure with these patients, I meet a great deal of resistance. They tell me, "Well, it's the only diet that ever worked for me." My obvious response is that it didn't work, because they're now right back where they started. Everyone wants fast results, and Atkins can give it to them. The only problem is that it's not a lasting result.

The South Beach Diet is based on the same principle as Atkins in that it recognizes the role that carbohydrates play in the dieting process, but the author (a physician) takes a much healthier approach: certain carbohydrates (primarily low-glycemic index carbs) are added into the high-protein diet early on in a graduated fashion. He also emphasizes the use of leaner and healthier types of protein. The only objection I really have to this diet is that you're eating a little differently every week, so you're not establishing those important routines right from the start. What I do like about the South Beach Diet is that most people, even after they've forsaken the diet, continue to eat far fewer sugar-laden and starchy carbs than they used to eat, and this is a very good thing.

What lessons can we take away from high-protein diets that will help us in our quest for a truly successful change in our habits? Exactly what are the tricks to eating more calories and getting away with it? Well, if you haven't already guessed, it's reducing certain types of carbohydrates in your diet. If you eat meals that are composed primarily of lean protein and nonstarchy vegetables, you can probably eat an extra 100 to 150 calories, or even more, in a meal and get away with it. Knowing that it is unrealistic to give up all the simple but comforting carbohydrates forever, let's establish a program that allows for those too.

When you have become accustomed to eating five meals a day, each of those meals can be modified according to not only what's available, but to what you feel like eating at any particular time. Remember when I said it is much easier to modify one of five meals as opposed to one of two? This aspect allows you the flexibility to actually stay with the plan and not break the rules.

So can an off-and-on low-carb system really work? I wouldn't be writing this book if it didn't. But please, make certain you have enough information to tailor this new system according to the principles you are presently following.

Think about the principle behind a low-carb meal, then apply this knowledge to your daily eating habits. When you eat only protein and fat and haven't eaten much in the carbohydrate family, your insulin levels remain low. Even though your body has begun to process these foods, without the insulin, the foods cannot enter the cells.

But how long do these nutrients hang around before your body eliminates them? As far as I know, that hasn't been studied, so it's a bit of guesswork. All we know is that they do hang around. So whenever you choose to eat a higher-calorie low-carb meal, you'll need to wait awhile (generally half-a-day) before eating any high-carb foods. Since very high-carb meals are not very filling (the higher the density, the smaller the volume), they will, by their very nature, become less frequent choices. However, what is important is that they will remain part of your overall diet plan.

So, from a practical standpoint, how does the above information fit into our diet scheme?

Suppose you wake up one Sunday morning with a tremendous craving for bacon, eggs, and sausage. That's fine; just stay away from muffins, bagels, bread, and pancakes. Keep those insulin levels down, and you won't absorb that much of your meal ... but choose your next meal carefully. Unlike dinner, your breakfast is followed by a meal only a few hours later. You need to be careful not to include many carbohydrates in your second meal. Also, keep that second meal on target in terms of calories; you don't want any extra calories floating in your bloodstream.

If you decide on a sandwich, make certain the bread is high-fiber, low-carb bread. Your fourth meal of the day is probably safe for higher carb content. (In other words, the two meals that follow an indulgent high-protein, low-carb meal need to also be low in carbs.)

Don't put a high-calorie, low-carb meal too close to a meal that includes a lot of carbohydrates!

Let's discuss a different scenario. Let's say that you are really doing well with the five or six small meals per day. Breakfast was a healthy 350 calories. Midmorning, you had a 350-calorie sandwich (or half a sandwich). At lunch, you ran out to get a few errands done, and you passed a bakery and couldn't resist. So instead of eating lunch, you had a piece of chocolate cake (a 350-calorie piece). Late afternoon or early evening, you ate the other half of your sandwich from lunch. And now it's dinnertime, and you'd really like to have a nice, juicy steak for dinner—a piece that's larger than 350 calories worth. Go ahead; it's okay as long as the steak is accompanied only by a salad or another low glycemic index food. You cannot eat a potato or rice with that steak, because then you'll absorb most of those plentiful calories. What's important to remember is that high caloric, high protein meals take time to be processed and will be totally absorbed if accompanied or followed by sufficient carbs. High-density carbs in the preceding meal will have no effect, since they have long since been digested.

This illustration shows you that you can eat all kinds of food and still stay with the plan. This on-again, off-again system will help you lose, and then maintain, your weight. I'm not recommending you eat chocolate cake or steak every day. What I am saying is that the occasional day like this is still within an acceptable range.

Since carbohydrates comprise so many different types of foods, it is important to classify them, so as to better understand how they can be used or not used in a low-carb diet. As we discussed, the original Atkins Diet allowed no carbs. That's easy to understand. Only protein and fat were allowed. In the revised Atkins Diet, some carbs are allowed, but which ones? The answer is the carbs that will have the least effect on your insulin levels. These tend to be low-density carbs. Stated another way, these foods have a low glycemic index.

Scientists figured out a way to measure the influence that foods have in raising blood-sugar levels. The more a certain food raises the sugar level in your bloodstream, the higher its GI (glycemic index). In the appendix of this book, you will find a more complete explanation and a general listing.

So make sure your low-carb meal includes only low-glycemic-index carbohydrates for accompaniment to any protein or fat you have chosen. These foods will, by their very nature, be low in calories. But beware: you can't eat as much as you want during these low-carb meals, because calories still matter. But for additional flexibility, these meals can have as much as 500 calories for women and 600 for men.

Hopefully, you now have a better understanding of how to fit a low-carb meal into your day.

Understanding these diet principles fully may take a little time, these very principles will give you the kind of flexibility you need to succeed.

Let's review our steps.

Step 1: Stop drinking your calories

Step 2: Eat breakfast

Step 3: Eat a small meal between breakfast and lunch

Step 4: Eat an appetizer a few hours before dinner

Step 5: Find exercise that you enjoy.

Step 6: (Part 1) Refine your meals to goal size through the low density method.

Step 6: (Part 2) Refine your meals to goal size through the high protein method.

Chapter Seventeen

March 2006

By the end of her trip home from Dr. Lang's office, Cheryl was very pensive. *How can I put some of this new information to work?* She liked Dr. Lang's suggestion of a weight vest; when she had an opportunity, she would get one. The desk-side exercises didn't really appeal to her, although she hadn't entirely given up on the idea. Doing Atkins two times a week seemed like a really promising idea. She remembered how well that particular diet had worked for her in the past, but she was leery of slowing her metabolism. She remembered how quickly she had gained the weight back after losing the fifty pounds.

"Mom, I'm home!" Cheryl announced as she walked in the door.

Charlotte was watching *Wheel of Fortune*. "I Love Lucy in the Sky with Diamonds!" she shouted at the screen. "Oh, hi, sweetheart. How was your doctor's appointment?"

"Pretty good. I was really frustrated that I'd only lost seven pounds this time, but I think I have a handle on it. Have you had anything to eat yet?"

"No, but I'm really not very hungry."

"You're never hungry. I don't know what it is with you, Ma. How are you ever going to get any better when you don't eat anything? You need to eat to build yourself up."

"I've been doing just fine. Just last week, the doctor told me I was doing really well. And thanks to your cooking, I actually gained two pounds. Funny, isn't it? You cook, and it sends us in opposite directions. Somebody should study that scientifically."

"Hey, no big mystery, Mom. Home cooking beats food in a cardboard box!"

"I couldn't agree more," said Charlotte. "So what are you making tonight?"

"I thought I'd make that spaghetti squash again. I have some leftover marinara sauce. It shouldn't take very long."

"That sounds good."

"I'll let you know when it's ready," Cheryl said on her way out to the kitchen. Her mother returned her attention to *Wheel of Fortune*.

"The Washington Monument!" Charlotte proclaimed. She was again solving the puzzles long before the contestants.

Cheryl continued to brood over that day's doctor visit. She was really beginning to understand what Dr. Lang had meant in their earlier conversations about how much there was to know about healthy eating and losing weight. It was really so much more complicated than anyone would think. *No wonder we all fail so miserably,* Cheryl thought. *Most of us really don't have a clue when we embark on a diet. Sure, when we were younger, losing weight was really easy, but boy oh boy, it's sure not so easy now. I wish I knew then what I know now. If I hadn't gone on that Atkins Diet and lost all that weight, I might still have that twenty-five pounds of muscle mass I'd lost.*

No sense crying over spilled milk, she admonished herself. *Onward and upward. I will* do this!

Cheryl decided she would do the Atkins thing on Mondays and Thursdays, when she wasn't going to the dance studio. She knew from previous experience that she might not have as much energy on those days.

As the weeks went by, Cheryl noticed something interesting about the day following the Atkins Diet. She seemed to lose an extra pound or two, but then it was right back on the following day. She realized it was the water weight that had disappeared temporarily. However, as the weeks passed, she did note that the weight was coming off a bit more rapidly.

Cheryl was amazed at how much harder the weight vest made her practice sessions. When she took it off, she felt as if she could float through the air; it was almost a mind-altering experience. All in all, she was very pleased with how she was progressing. After six weeks, she had lost another six pounds—almost as much as in the previous three months combined. Everything was perfect; she was right on track.

Well, everything is almost perfect—but everything would be perfect if Victor would just ask me out on a date already. She saw him regularly, and he was always polite and charming, but the date never seemed to happen.

At least he had started talking to her a little more. At each dance party, she learned something new about him. She found out that he was really interested in computers and wasn't all that happy with dance instruction, but he was obligated to help his mom at the studio. Another evening, Cheryl learned more about his dad—that he lived in Florida and worked for NASA. Victor's family, she learned, had traveled around a lot when he was a kid, because his father was always changing jobs. It wasn't until his parents divorced that Victor settled in Philadelphia with his mother. At another dance party, she was surprised to find out that he had gone to Temple University and actually had a degree in computer science, and that it was the first time he had spent more than two years in any one city. He was happy staying put. The only thing he regretted was that he had rarely gotten to see his dad since the divorce; he really missed his father. His dad was the one who had gotten him interested in computers in the first place.

Cheryl commiserated with Victor's loss. She had lost her dad, and she knew what that felt like. At least Victor's dad was alive ... but she wondered if that wasn't even worse. Victor's dad could come back, but he didn't.

But still, Victor didn't ask her out. Maybe he was just being nice, putting his best foot forward as an emissary of the dance studio, doing his duty by making the customers happy. Somehow, though, Cheryl didn't think so. He didn't seem to share his past with anyone else, so maybe he was interested. Cheryl pondered what she could do. Should she actually ask him out? Maybe she'd work up the courage. She ran through all kinds of possible approaches in her mind, but they all sounded awkward and contrived. She just couldn't find the nerve ... maybe next week. She'd discuss it with Teresa. Maybe Teresa would have some ideas.

That Monday, the two women both managed to get a few extra minutes for lunch, so Cheryl suggested they meet at O'Neal's. It was a local bar, but she loved their hamburgers. As they ordered lunch, Teresa was a bit surprised to see Cheryl order a cheeseburger.

"What gives?" Teresa asked. "Where's the new Cheryl, who never would have suggested this restaurant in the first place?"

Cheryl's quick explanation that seemed to confuse Teresa more than anything. *I really have learned a lot*, Cheryl thought. *It's amazing how far I've come.* She changed the subject by mentioning her dilemma about Victor. She was pretty sure by now that Victor was interested in her, but she just didn't know what to do about it. Teresa concurred about Victor's interest. In fact, she said, she was surprised that they hadn't gotten together before now. She had told Cheryl on numerous occasions that Victor was surely attracted to her. Cheryl wanted to take the initiative, but she just didn't know how. Did Teresa have any ideas?

"I guess you could try another party," Teresa offered.

"Yeah, that worked real well the last time," Cheryl responded. "No, I want to go on a date with Victor. I just don't have the nerve to ask outright."

"What about mentioning that you'd like to see a certain movie? He might pick up on that and ask you to go with him."

"Actually, I tried that in the past, but he had already seen the movie, and just agreed I should go see it—that it was really good."

"Hmmm, let me think. What if you got tickets to something and asked him to join you? Oh, I know: pretend that someone gave you free tickets, like to a concert or something, and you don't have anyone to go with, because all your girlfriends are busy," Teresa said excitedly.

"That's a really great idea. I could do that," Cheryl responded, equally as excited.

Just then, their food came.

"Okay," Teresa said slowly, "Explain this whole cheeseburger thing to me again, will you?"

"Well, like I said, today's my Atkins day."

"You mentioned that, but I thought the doctor didn't want you to do any dieting." Teresa was clearly very curious now.

"I'm not exactly dieting," Cheryl explained as she took the cheeseburger off the roll and started eating it with a knife and a fork. She eschewed the potato salad that came with it, shoving it away from her to the other side of the table. "Dr. Lang explained that the problem with most diets is that they don't ingrain habits that you can live with for the rest of your life, and I certainly couldn't live with Atkins for a lifetime, but she did explain that there was no reason I couldn't use the principles of the diet to my advantage."

"I'm still not getting this," Teresa said with her mouth half full.

"Well, perhaps I didn't explain it well enough earlier. If I only do Atkins two days a week, it won't affect my already established good habits. More importantly, it won't slow down my metabolism the way it did the last time, especially if I keep up my dancing. That way, I can lose additional weight a little faster. She emphasized that I should eat a regular breakfast on those days and just do the Atkins thing the rest of the day, essentially eliminating the rest of the calories for that day."

"But how does it eliminate those calories?" Teresa was still a bit confused.

"Eating just protein and fat without any carbohydrates doesn't stimulate your insulin levels to rise, so you're unable to absorb the calories that you ate, and then your body eventually gets rid of them." Again, Cheryl was surprising herself by how much she was really learning about nutrition.

"That's really interesting. So why does she tell you to eat a regular breakfast on those days?" Teresa asked.

"Because you always want to break fast. I think she said that if you eat breakfast each morning and jump start your metabolism, you actually burn 300 more calories in the day than if you don't eat breakfast. The object is to try to eliminate more calories without slowing up your metabolism any further, so eating those calories in the morning is important to get things going."

"You know, that really is fascinating. How'd you learn all that stuff?"

"Dr. Lang's been teaching me, and she gives me chapters of her book to read. I didn't believe her in the beginning, when she had told me that most people don't succeed at dieting because they don't have enough information. I'm beginning to really appreciate how much I need to know to do this right. Applying that knowledge to my life hasn't always been the easiest thing in the world, but I'm really beginning to get it. I know I'm not there yet, but for the first time in fifteen years, I truly believe that I can be thin again … and stay thin."

"I'm so thrilled for you!" Teresa exclaimed. "You really seem to be figuring it out. So … getting back to Victor, what kind of tickets do you think would entice him to join you?"

"Probably to a computer show at the convention enter or some such thing, but why would I have tickets for a computer show? No, I think maybe a Broadway show … maybe a show with some dancing."

"How about *Mama Mia*? You could find out what nights he's usually free. After you make sure tickets are available but before you buy them, tell him you have them, and see what he says. If he agrees, you can buy the tickets later."

"That's such a great idea! Oh, gosh … look at the time. We'd better go. I have to get back to work." They paid the check in a hurry, and Cheryl practically ran the couple of blocks back to work.

The rest of the afternoon went smoothly. Cheryl was in a wonderful mood. She was sure that Victor would agree to come to a show with her; it was the perfect solution.

Soon, everything in her life would be perfect. If she could just keep on track for about another year, she'd be thin again. *Wow … who would have ever thought?*

Knowledge is important.

Putting it to appropriate use is even more so.

Can you, like Cheryl, relate what you've learned in a practical way?

STEP 7: APPLYING NEW KNOWLEDGE TO EVERYDAY MEALS

By
Nikki Lang, MD

Let's focus on how to apply the information we've learned so far to various situations.

1. Making dinner for the whole family.
2. Forgetting to take something out of the freezer.
3. Eating out at restaurants.
4. Going to parties.

Initially in this pursuit of dietary change, I encouraged eating five small meals a day and avoiding drinking your calories. Then I gave you a calorie guideline for those meals so that when you established new meals, you wouldn't have to change them a few weeks later to reflect that caloric range. I asked you to educate yourself with regard to calorie count by looking at nutritional panels, as well as looking foods up in a calorie-counting book. However, up until now, I haven't insisted that every single meal be within guidelines.

Beginning sometime in the second or third month, I'd like you to pick the meal that is giving you the most difficulty and focus on bringing that single meal to the proper calorie count. You can do it one of two ways. You can add 100 to 150 calories to the requirement and go low-carb, or you can focus on loading up with low-density foods.

Humans are creatures of habit. Once you find a meal that fits the bill, repeating it often will ultimately make it more desirable. So all you need to do is find six to eight meals that you really like, then repeat them often enough that you crave those meals.

I'm going to assume that dinner is usually the most difficult meal. Because dinner is usually the largest meal of the day, other obstacles might be in the way besides appetite. By having the fourth meal of the day a few hours before, you may have quelled most of your hunger, but you might have a family or partner to feed. Perhaps dinner is typically a social activity in your household, and you are accustomed to taking your time and eating a longer, more relaxing meal.

Let's discuss some possibilities. Let's say you just made fried chicken, potatoes, corn, and greens for your family. There is no reason why you couldn't have a small portion of the same chicken, lots of greens, and perhaps a salad. You would skip the corn and potatoes; remember, you wouldn't really be that hungry.

But perhaps you had a real craving for potatoes and just couldn't resist. In that case, you could always just skip the chicken, saving it for another meal. **Just because you're cooking for others, doesn't mean you have to eat everything yourself.**

Suppose you've forgotten to take something out of the freezer for dinner. If you keep items individually frozen (See chapter seven, "Other Habits That Need Changing That Maybe You Haven't Thought About"), then a careful defrost in the microwave will only take a few (five to ten) minutes. Or check out your cupboards. Have some pasta lurking there? An entire cup of cooked spaghetti is about 185 calories. Sauté a handful of vegetables (frozen or fresh), onions, mushrooms (50 calories), and garlic (or garlic powder, if that's all that's in the cupboard) in a tablespoon of olive oil (100 calories), or butter (Smart Balance for the cholesterol conscious) with the spaghetti. You now have a nice dish of vegetable pasta at 335 calories. You still have room for a salad, if you use a low-calorie dressing or just plain vinegar and lemon juice.

You're at a restaurant and want to stick to your plan, but you aren't sure how—the menu doesn't include calorie information. One of two methods might work for you. Either go with the low-carb meal and order the entrée, but ask them to leave the potatoes or pasta off and double up on the green vegetable, or ask for a doggie bag up front (or an extra plate if you're too embarrassed—your butter plate might work for this) and put half your meal aside before you even start eating. That way, you won't inadvertently eat too much while you're busy conversing over dinner.

Then, if you haven't already, load the rest into your doggie bag as another meal. Another way to deal with restaurant eating is to order two or three appetizers—depending, of course, on what they are.

Appetizers come in much smaller portions, and they sometimes give you an opportunity to taste a number of different foods without overeating. You still have to be careful of content, though. Let's say you've chosen to have soup, a Caesar salad, and clams casino. If the soup isn't a really rich, creamy soup (like lobster bisque, at 320 calories per cup), that combination will work. If the soup is creamy, you could eat only half of it, though I admit it's kind of hard to take leftover soup home. However, if you're not too embarrassed, you could say to the waitress halfway through, "Is there any way I could take the rest of this soup home? It's absolutely delicious, but I just can't finish it."

Perhaps you've gone to an ethnic restaurant—Chinese, Thai, or Indian. Ordering several different appetizers is a great way to taste different things without eating too much. Of course, sharing entrées is common in these types of restaurants. Just remember to exercise caution; if you do order too much, plan what you're going to take home before you finish eating, so you don't overeat.

Speaking of sharing, I know a couple who are somewhat older and really enjoy going out to eat, but do not have the capacity to eat the large quantities offered at most restaurants. They usually decide on a mutual appetizer and main entrée, then share both. This is another strategy if you are eating out with someone who also wishes to keep his or her meals smaller.

Suppose you're not at a restaurant, but at a party or family barbecue. How can you stay on track then? Consider several factors. First of all, how long are you going to be there? More than three hours? Then guess what? You can eat twice! Survey what food is being served. Is anything there you absolutely have to have? That's going to dictate which direction you need to go.

If the one food you must have is a protein, then you may want to go with low-carb meals for the day, but be sure to avoid any starches or other higher-glycemic-index foods. On the other hand, even if you do want some protein, you may choose to go with the low-calorie option, so you'll be able to eat a little starch or dessert. If it's potatoes you crave, you'll want to go with a calorie limitation. But remember, you need to keep your protein and fat portions small if you're eating both. The best part is that you get to eat twice!

Need a little more rigidity to the plan in the beginning? Then eat your 350 calories at the beginning of the party and again toward the end of the party. Let's say you're at a barbecue, and you'd like to have a hamburger on a roll. Well, that's really all you can afford to eat for the first meal, except for maybe some salad (the lettuce type, not the pasta type), but later you can eat your potato or macaroni salad or other higher glycemic foods. Just keep tabs on your calories. The other possibility is to eat only the hamburger without the roll, and then dig into the salad or other low-glycemic foods; or eat several hamburgers, hot dogs, or pieces of chicken, and then just stay away from the carbs. It's all doable—it just requires a bit of educated balance.

Another possibility is just to nibble your way through the party. Eat a little, chat with friends, and then eat a little more while you continue your conversations. Keep the portions small. Interestingly, by doing this, you actually markedly reduce your appetite (just like having that appetizer before dinner and waiting) and really won't want much more. Is this liable to happen in the beginning of this program? Not really, because you haven't yet truly acquired the habit of frequent, smaller meals. But don't let this bother you—the real key is what you do over the long term, not what happens once a month.

If you end up eating too much at the party, just regroup and start again the next day with the program. You can work on the party thing next time.

A recent experience I had, which was good for my eating habits but a little embarrassing socially, will serve to illustrate my point. I was at a dinner party. When we sat down at the table, I saw appetizers spread out across the table that included different types of Italian meats, cheeses, olives, peppers, and other condiments. I took a little of each. Following this, the hostess served us some delicious ravioli stuffed with various ingredients. I ate two or three of these (they were the large ravioli). More than satisfied, I was startled to realize that dinner was yet to come! Suddenly, roasted meat, potatoes, and several vegetables appeared on the table, followed by salad. I had to apologize to my hostess, as I was absolutely unable to eat another thing.

That was not discipline on my part. My stomach is so accustomed to smaller meals that it screams at me if I try to eat a larger one.

Repetition over time remains the key. Although you may encounter many obstacles that will make it difficult to eat those five small meals, a little thought on your part will allow you to figure out how to accommodate each situation. Take pride in your successes, and repeat them often. Renew your determination after any failures, and figure out how to avoid them.

Let's review our steps.

Step 1: **Stop drinking your calories**

Step 2: **Eat breakfast**

Step 3: **Eat a small meal between breakfast and lunch**

Step 4: **Eat an appetizer a few hours before dinner**

Step 5: **Find exercise that you enjoy.**

Step 6: **(Part 1) Refine your meals to goal size through the low density method.**

Step 6: **(Part 2) Refine your meals to goal size through the high protein method.**

Step 7: **Apply your new-found knowledge to everyday meals.**

Unlike Cheryl, you may find the Desk-Side Exercise Program helpful.

DESK-SIDE EXERCISE PROGRAM
By
Nikki Lang, MD

I have compiled a bunch of exercises you can do at your desk at work, or at home. These aren't designed to serve as your only exercise, but they can help you make progress even as you're still deciding on an exercise routine, or augment the routine you already have.

These exercises work the upper body, torso, and lower body. You can rotate through the exercises, doing upper body one day, torso the next, and lower body the third day, then repeating the cycle. You don't need to do all the exercises at once; do a few from one category at a time throughout the day.

As you become familiar with the exercises, they will, of course, take a lot less time. None of them are difficult, but some of them will probably make you more sore than you bargained for, because they work muscles that you don't often engage. These exercises do not take the place of more vigorous exercise, but they are far superior to no exercise.

UPPER BODY

Exercise 1

Sit in your office chair with your back straight, elevate your arms out to the sides, and bend your elbows at right angles so that your fingers are pointing at the ceiling and your thumbs are toward each other. Make certain that your upper arms are level with your shoulders. Keeping your elbows level with your shoulders and your fingers perpendicular to the ceiling, move your arms backward in an attempt to touch the back of your chair. You will only be able to move a few inches, but you will feel tension between your shoulder blades. Hold for 3 counts before returning to the start position. Repeat 10 times.

Exercise 2

Hold your arms out to the sides, elbows straight, palms facing the floor, and thumbs straight ahead. Attempt to touch the ceiling. Again, you will only be able to move several inches; don't allow your arms to drift forward or rotate slightly. Remember, your thumbs are straight ahead, your palms are parallel to the floor, and your arms are even with the rest of your body, not in front of it. Again, hold for 3 counts before returning to the starting position and repeating 10 times.

Exercise 3

Now, while still holding your arms out to your sides, bend your elbows down so that your fingers are pointing toward the floor and your palms are facing backward. This time, lift your elbows as high as you can, hold for 3 counts, and return to the starting position. Repeat 10 times.

Exercise 4

Place your palms together in front of your chest, with your elbows elevated out to the sides. Press your palms together as hard as you can, and hold for 10 counts. Repeat 10 times.

Exercise 5

Hold a heavy book, or other manageable object, in one hand, much the same way a waiter might hold a tray full of dishes. Your arm should be out to the side, elbow bent at a 90-degree angle, forearm parallel to the plane of your body. Raise the object slowly until your arm is straight, then slowly lower it back. Repeat 10 times, then switch arms and repeat. Pick heavier objects as you improve. (You may want to bring a small barbell into work and keep it in a drawer.)

Exercise 6

Sitting up as tall as possible, grab the edge of your desk with both hands, using an underhand grip. Make sure that you're far enough away from your desk so that your elbows are only slightly bent. Pull yourself in toward

your desk as far as you can, then press outward, straightening your arms to move yourself away from your desk and
back to the starting position. Repeat 10 times. If your
chair does not have wheels, then begin with your arms bent
a little more than 90 degrees. Plant your feet onto the
floor and just pull on the desk for 3 slow counts. Pull as
if you were trying to move it toward you, then push on it
for another 3 slow counts, and repeat the cycle 10 times.

Exercise 7
Repeat the same exercise as above, but grab the desk
with an overhand grip.

Exercise 8
Stand about an arm's length away from a wall, with your
palms pressed against it and your feet about hip width
apart. Bend your elbows, and let your body move toward
the wall. Once your elbows are bent to about 90 degrees,
straighten your arms and return to the start.

If you are able, stand a few feet away from your desk,
then put your hands on the edge of the desk, shoulder width
apart. Keep your back straight; your shoulders, hips, and
ankles should be in a straight line. Hold your abdominal muscles tight and lower your chest toward the desk by
bending your elbows as far as you are able, then push back
up slowly.

Repeat either of the above 10 times.

Exercise 9
Stand with your back to the desk about one or two feet
away. Place your hands, palms down, on the desktop behind
you. Cross one leg over the other. Bend your arms and
lower yourself toward the floor—using your legs for support, but bending your knees as you move toward the floor.
Push yourself up by straightening your arms, not pushing
up with your legs. And—you guessed it—repeat 10 times.

Exercise 10
While sitting, put your palms on the arms of the chair,
push down, and begin straightening your arms until your
butt is raised up off the chair. Slowly return to a sit-

ting position. If your chair has no arms, then place your palms on the seat of the chair and try to lift your butt of the seat, and then slowly relax. Again, repeat 10 times.

TORSO

Exercise 1

While sitting upright, breathe in, expanding your abdomen and chest. On the exhale, contract your abdominal muscles, moving your navel toward your spine, and simultaneously press your inner thighs and knees together. Maintain the contraction in your abdominal and inner thigh muscles for five to six seconds while you exhale fully and completely. Repeat 5 times.

Exercise 2

Stand straight up from your chair, taking care not to lock your knees into a full straightened position or over-arch your lower back. As you do so, contract (or "squeeze") your buttocks. At the top of the motion, squeeze the buttocks even tighter, and slowly sit back down, touching your buttocks only lightly to the chair before you stand back up into the next repetition. Repeat 5 times. (Alternatively, consider doing this as many times per day as you stand up. Or, when you take a phone call, incorporate a squat at the beginning, middle, and end of the call.)

Exercise 3

Sit tall, with one hand behind your head and the other one holding onto the side edge of your seat. Pull your abdominal muscles inward. Slowly curl down and forward just a few inches. As you do so, pull your abs in even tighter. Hold a moment, then slowly uncurl to a very tall position. Again, repeat 5 times. These are similar to crunches, but performed vertically.

Exercise 4

Sitting in your swivel chair, holding onto your desk, turn your waist as far as you can to each side. Sit somewhat close to the edge of the chair so that you can reach out to hold onto your desk. Then twist without your legs impeding your motion. Repeat 10 times slowly in each direction.

Exercise 5

Sit up straight, with your weight evenly distributed on both buttocks. Breathe in, and relax your shoulders. Breathe out, and draw in the pelvic-floor muscles, as if you are preventing yourself from having a bowel movement. You should feel no tension in your stomach. Breathe in, and relax everything but the buttock muscles; breathe out, and continue to draw up the pelvic floor. Extend this contraction into the lower abdominals. You should feel tension to the belly button only. Breathe in, and completely relax in the reverse direction. Now breathe out, draw in the pelvic floor, and continue up the whole abdominal muscle, as if you are bracing for a punch. Now breathe in and relax downward, maintaining the tension solely in your buttocks. Repeat the whole cycle 5 times.

Exercise 6

While holding onto your chair for balance, extend both legs as if you were sitting on the floor, toes pointing toward the ceiling. Pull your heels toward your body and bend your knees, trying to keep your heels level with the seat of your chair. Keep your knees fully bent for 3 counts. Slowly stretch your legs straight ahead without lowering them to the floor. Repeat 10 times, or as many times as you are able.

Exercise 7

Slide forward in your seat to only about two to three inches from the edge. Wrap your feet around the legs of the chair or under your desk. (This is for balance, to counter the backward movement.) Now stretch your arms straight up in the air, arching your back. Lean back very slowly until you lightly touch the back of your chair with your upper back, but do not use the chair back for support. Hold that position for as long as you possibly can, then return to the starting position. You only need to do this exercise once, but each time, you should try to hold it longer and longer—up to two or three minutes if possible.

LOWER BODY

Exercise 1

In a standing position, slowly bend your knees until your body is three quarters of the way down to the floor. While remaining in this semi-squat, move up four inches and back down again 10 times. Hold onto your desk for balance.

Exercise 2

Do the same as above, except squat down as far as possible without resting on the lower portion of your leg. From that position, move through the same small range of four inches. Repeat 10 times.

Exercise 3

Stand up, face your desk, and hold on for balance. Lift up your left leg and rest your left foot behind your right calf. Slowly raise yourself up on your toes, then slowly lower yourself back down. Repeat 10 times. Switch feet and repeat.

Exercise 4

Holding onto your desk with one hand if necessary, lift your toes off the floor and walk around your desk on your heels 5 times. If your desk is against a wall, walk back and forth in front of the desk 10 times.

Exercise 5

Now sit in your chair, turning it away from your desk so you can extend one of your legs directly in front of you, foot flexed with toes toward the ceiling. Slowly move your leg outward, holding your leg level with your other knee. Move outward as far as you can, or as far as your chair will allow. Hold your leg in that position for 3 counts, then slowly return to the start position straight in front of you. Repeat 3 times, then start over. Swing your chair around to the opposite side and repeat above with the other leg.

Exercise 6

Stand facing your desk. Put your palms down on the desktop for support. Extend one leg out behind you. Keep your leg straight, and raise it as high as possible. Lower your leg slowly; don't rush. Repeat 10 times, then start over with the other leg.

Exercise 7

Now, while still standing, extend one leg directly out to the side as far as you can. Hold it for a count of three, then slowly lower your leg. Repeat 10 times, then switch legs and start over.

No matter which form of exercise you choose, just make certain that you choose something. No matter how small that change is, it's still better than doing nothing.

Remember, little changes add up!

Chapter Eighteen

May 2006

Cheryl arrived home, eager to share Teresa's dating scheme with her mom. Those thoughts evaporated as soon as she saw her mom on a stretcher on the way out the front door of her house.

"Oh, Mommmm," she wailed. "I'm just not ready for you to die. Not now ... please, not yet." She ran to the side of the stretcher and picked up Charlotte's free hand. "Oh, God, please not yet. Mom, please wake up. I need you ... please. I need you so much."

One of the paramedics, who had been squeezing the breathing bag with one hand and pushing the stretcher with the other, spoke to Cheryl calmly but firmly. "You can ride with us, miss, but please let us do our job. Please step aside so we can get her in the ambulance as quickly as possible."

Cheryl let go of her mother's hand and stood back. Tears flowed down her face. Mollie came over and put her arms around her.

"Oh, Mrs. Curtis, what am I going to do? What if she dies? I don't know how I'm going to do anything without her. Oh, God, please don't let her die!"

"Miss?" The same paramedic was motioning for her to get inside the ambulance.

"That's okay," Cheryl answered. "I'll follow in my car." She turned to Mollie. "Would you come to the hospital with me?"

"Of course, dear. Just give me time to grab my purse and a sweater. I'll be back in a jiffy."

When they arrived at the hospital's emergency room, they were forced to wait in the waiting room as the doctors were "working on" Cheryl's mother. *Do I even want to know what that means?* Cheryl thought, as shock spread through her body.

Cheryl would alternately pace up and down, then sit next to Mollie and hold her hands and cry quietly. She just knew that something was different this time—and not in a good way. She kept praying to herself that her mother would pull through, but dreaded the worst.

"I'm so sorry, Cheryl," Mollie said. "I shouldn't have left Charlotte alone. I should have stayed with her. It's all my fault."

"Your fault ... how could it be your fault? You didn't make her ill."

"Well, after our card game, she wasn't feeling so well. She said that it was the chicken salad ... that it was too spicy. I wanted to call her doctor, but she wouldn't let me."

"So, you see, it couldn't be your fault," Cheryl concluded. "Mom wouldn't let you call the doctor."

"But I should have stayed with her, Cheryl. She didn't look so good. But she said she just wanted to lie down and rest."

"Oh, Mrs. Curtis, you've known my mother longer than I have. Have you ever really known her not to get her way?" Cheryl actually had the tiniest bit of a smile on her face.

Mollie half smiled back. "No, you're right: she always manages to do what she wants to do. I'm just really grateful that I decided to go back and check on her.

"So am I," Cheryl responded.

They both became silent again.

It seemed like hours before anyone came out to talk to them. The news was both good and bad. Charlotte had had a heart attack. But since it had only been hours old, the doctors had been able to break up the clot. She was now stable and remained unconscious, but they didn't know if there was any brain damage. She was, of course, on a respirator. They were going to transfer her to the ICU shortly, and both Cheryl and Mollie could see her there once she was settled in.

"Do you know how long it will be before we can see her?" Cheryl asked.

"She's on her way up now, so I would say in about thirty-five or forty minutes," the ER doctor responded.

"Thank you, Doctor," Mollie said. "Thank you for all your help."

It was getting late, and neither Cheryl nor Mollie had had any dinner. Mollie tried to persuade Cheryl to go to the cafeteria to get something to eat.

"I'm not hungry. I couldn't eat a thing." Cheryl began pacing again, not knowing what else to do.

"You may not be hungry, my dear, but this little old lady is starving, and if I don't get something to eat, I'll pass out. We don't need to put another patient in this hospital today!"

"Oh, Mrs. Curtis, I'm so sorry. I've been so wrapped up in myself that I didn't consider how you must be feeling. Please forgive me. Of course we should go to the cafeteria."

Cheryl broke down and got a turkey sandwich, but in the end, she only ate a couple of bites. Mollie, bless her soul, ate every last bit of chicken cacciatore and rice off her plate.

Cheryl was silent most of the time, as was Mollie. Finally, Cheryl broke the silence. "What am I going to do without her?" she asked, not really expecting a response.

"Why don't you cross that bridge when you come to it? She might pull through, and all this worry will be for naught."

"But what if they can't get her off the respirator? She was lucky the last time, but she'd only stopped taking some of her meds. Now, after a heart attack … they might never get her off that machine. What will I do then?"

"Cheryl, Cheryl, Cheryl. Stop worrying about what might be. It isn't useful. You know, years ago, a friend of mine once gave me some very sage advice about worrying, and I'm going to pass it on to you. She said, 'If there's a problem, and you can do something about it, don't worry—just do it! And if there's nothing you can possibly do about something, then what's the point of worrying? It's out of your hands anyway.'"

"That's so easy to say, but not easy to do."

"I know, honey, but try it. For now, just try to stay in the present. Don't think about what might be; just focus on what is. Your mom is still alive, and she has a fighting chance. Let's pray for her. Before we go to the ICU, would you like to go to the chapel with me?"

Cheryl hadn't been in church for years—not since Joy died. She wasn't sure whether it was from guilt that she had let God down by failing to protect her sister or from anger that God had let her down by failing to do the same thing. She had attempted to go on several occasions, but just couldn't get across the threshold of the church. Somehow, she thought it would be hypocritical. She wasn't even sure that she still believed in God.

Cheryl shook her head, so Mollie told Cheryl that she would catch up with her in the ICU waiting room and went to the chapel by herself.

When Cheryl finally got to see her mother, she was surprised. Charlotte looked pretty good, considering. Her color was the best Cheryl had seen in a long time. She appeared to be resting very comfortably. Cheryl took her mother's hand and just sat quietly by the bedside for a while. She was frightened, but in an attempt at normalcy, she started talking to her mom as though she had just gotten home from work. She told Charlotte of her plans to invite Victor to a show. She talked about all types of mundane things, but mostly about how much she needed and loved her mother.

Cheryl finally stopped talking and just sat and held Charlotte's hand for a while. To Cheryl's surprise, the nurses let Mollie come in. Mollie explained that she had known that only close relatives were allowed in the ICU, so she had told the doctors she was Charlotte's sister. It was late, and everything was very quiet, and since this was the first day of Charlotte's admission, the doctors allowed more than one visitor in the room. Mollie agreed with Cheryl that Charlotte looked really good.

By the time they had finally left the hospital at about one in the morning, they were both a little bit optimistic that Charlotte might pull through.

Several days passed, but Charlotte failed to wake up. Cheryl had called out of work and spent most days by her bedside, waiting for her to open her eyes and listening to the hiss of the respirator. Cheryl talked to her as if nothing were wrong and read aloud to her from some of her favorite books. When that didn't work, Cheryl pleaded with her to get better. She tried everything. She even started going to the chapel, figuring that a little praying couldn't hurt either.

All of Charlotte's friends pitched in to help Cheryl. They brought all kinds of food, so she wouldn't have to cook. They spent hours with her, trying to reassure her—but to no avail. As each day went by and her mother failed to improve, Cheryl became more and more distraught and depressed.

She regressed to old habits, reminiscent of the sleepless nights she had spent after Joy had disappeared from her life. She began eating mindlessly while staring at the TV, not really seeing. Dishes started piling up in the sink. The place might've turned into a real pigsty if it hadn't been for all of her mother's friends, as well as her own.

Mollie Curtis, Anna O'Hara, and Maggie Spencer all pitched in to help. They took turns cleaning and cooking and keeping her company. Teresa came by regularly. Susan, Wendy, and Carol pitched in as well, though they had somewhat more demanding schedules due to their family obligations.

With each passing day that her mother remained in a coma, Cheryl became less and less animated until she seemed like a zombie, going through the motions of life but not really living.

After Cheryl had spent two weeks in this zombielike state, Teresa finally managed to drag her to the doctor. She went in the room with Cheryl to make sure that Dr. Lang got the full story.

"Talk to me, Cheryl," Dr. Lang said gently. "I can't help you if you don't let me know what's bothering you."

Cheryl looked at her and just started crying.

Dr. Lang had been told about the situation with her mother, and she was aware how close they were.

"Are you sleeping?" she asked. Cheryl shook her head.

"You know, Cheryl, when we experience tremendous stress, our brain's chemistry dramatically shifts. It's one of the reasons you're having trouble sleeping. What I'd like to do is prescribe an antidepressant to begin helping your brain to shift its chemistry back to normal. It will only be temporary, but I think if we can help you get a good night's sleep, your days will become a little easier to handle.

"When was the last time you ate? We haven't done any blood work in a while, and I'd like to see how you're doing."

"I don't think she's eaten yet today, Doc," Teresa answered. "I'm afraid she hasn't been doing too well in that department lately."

"Then I guess we can take her blood. I see that her weight is two pounds less than the last visit, so she can't have fallen off the wagon too hard."

"Well, she had lost an additional six or seven pounds since she last saw you, but I guess she's put some of it back on. That's no surprise, the way she's been eating. I will say this, though: she really doesn't chow on any junk food to speak of, and she drinks all diet soda and water now. Most of the food she has in the house is pretty healthy. I guess that's why she hasn't gained that much back."

"That's why changing habits works. Anyway, I'd like to see Cheryl back in two weeks. Hold on just a sec." Dr. Lang stepped out of the exam room and returned shortly with some samples of an antidepressant. She handed them to Cheryl. "Just take one each morning and let me see you back here in two weeks. Okay?"

Cheryl nodded her response and got up to leave.

"No, don't leave yet. I want Latisha to take your blood."

Cheryl sat back down. Teresa put her arm around her silent friend. "Thanks, Doc. I really appreciate your help," Teresa said.

"Don't hesitate to call before the two weeks is up if the pills aren't helping. She does need to get some sleep."

"I will," Teresa answered.

The antidepressant did begin to help. Cheryl began sleeping better, and her days were not so muted. She felt a little more alive, and just in time: her office called and wanted to know when she could come back to work. They needed her desperately. She resolved to go back to work the following week. It would probably do her some good to occupy her time and her mind. Certainly, fretting constantly over her mother was not helping.

She started eating better again, since her sleeping patterns had improved. But she just couldn't seem to get motivated to do any exercise. She was in no mood to dance.

She began doing her own shopping and cooking again. In fact, having so much time on her hands, she decided she would try some new recipes with some new vegetables. She was getting really tired of the same old ones all the time. Her vegetable repertoire was rather meager, as there weren't many that she liked. The only new one she'd had up until now was the spaghetti squash.

She suddenly remembered that Dr. Lang had once given her a chapter about learning to like vegetables. She hoped she still had it after all this time. She flipped through the pages, which she now kept in one place on her desk, and found the chapter. She read the text with interest. She realized it simply took the principles she already knew about acquired taste and applied them to vegetables. She decided to buy a zucchini and cook it, as was suggested, in onions and garlic. How could it be bad? She loved onions and garlic.

Thank goodness, I'm finally starting to get back on track. Maybe going back to work was a good idea. She thought of Mrs. Curtis's admonishment not to worry about things you have no control over. She'd just try to be as patient as she could while waiting for her mother to wake up.

Do you, like Cheryl, eat few vegetables?
Read the following chapter and learn how to like more.
It's an important part of creating satisfying, low-calorie meals!

HOW DO I LEARN TO LIKE VEGETABLES?
By
Nikki Lang, MD

By now, you have begun to realize just how important vegetables are in the process of eating healthy. They provide important bulk to your diet, as well as variety and interest. If you want to be able to sit down to a low-calorie meal that is fully satisfying, vegetables really need to be an intrinsic part of your diet.

If you don't like vegetables or like very few vegetables, you really need to work at increasing the variety of vegetables in your diet. How do you go about that as painlessly as possible?

In the first few chapters, we discussed the importance of acquired taste and how to go about acquiring a taste for diet soda. Developing a taste for vegetables works basically the same way. You need to blindside your taste buds in a similar fashion. Let's start with some simple suggestions. Most people like garlic and fried onions, which are very pungent and have overwhelming flavors. Most anything that you cook with them will also taste like onions and garlic. So my first suggestion is to take any vegetable of which you are not terribly fond, cut it up into smaller bite-size pieces, and sauté it with onions and garlic. Garlic powder will work just fine, or minced garlic you buy in a jar. Use as much garlic and onions as it takes to make the dish palatable to you.

Each time you make this vegetable dish, you should use slightly less garlic and slightly less onion. Slowly, the vegetable flavor will peek through. The more familiar your palate gets with that vegetable, the less offensive it will become. In fact, believe it or not, you'll even begin to like it. Eventually, you'll be able to eat the vegetable without the onions and garlic and actually enjoy it.

What do you do if you don't like onions or garlic? Well, this plan will work equally well with just one of the two, or some other combination of ingredients that disguises the taste. I would suggest, however, also gradually learning to acquire a taste for both onions and garlic by using the powdered form. Sprinkle one or the other on foods that you do like to begin acquiring a taste for them. They are wonderful additions to any diet repertoire.

Do you like curry? You can use curry powder to season vegetables. If you don't know what curry is, then try something else. Barbecue sauce would work as well. Just make sure you cook the vegetable long enough in the sauce to pick up the flavor. It's important to cut the vegetable into small pieces in the beginning so that more sides are coated with your preferred flavor. As you become more accustomed to the flavor of the vegetable, you can make the pieces larger.

Another method is to put the vegetables into soups and stews. Again, keep the pieces small. You can make a mini chicken stew by sautéing small chunks of chicken (about 2 ounces) with onions, mushrooms (if you like mushrooms), and about 3/4 to 1 cup of mixed vegetables (from a bag of frozen mixed vegetables) for about 5 to 7 minutes, and then add 1/2 can cream of mushroom soup. Simmer for about another 5 minutes, and then enjoy your single portion of "chicken mushroom stew." The vegetables should be sufficiently disguised.

I don't know if you've ever picked up any powdered soups at the supermarket, but they get fancier and more interesting by the day. Recently, I found a hot-and-sour soup in powder form. You can take one vegetable, cut it in small pieces, cook it in the microwave for 2 minutes, and then add it to the heated soup, along with one raw egg. (The raw egg cooks in the hot soup.) This is another tasty way to sneak in those vegetables. Of course, you'll still have to repeat the experience many times to slowly acquire a taste for the vegetable. Once you find it okay in a more flavorful soup like this one, then you can try it in a more bland chicken soup that allows more vegetable flavor to peek through. More and more exposure will adjust your palate to that particular flavor.

Vegetable casseroles are another great place for vegetables to hide. You can find hundreds of recipes on the Internet. Just put the name of the vegetable in the search box and up comes hundreds, if not thousands, of possibilities. Keep looking until you find a recipe that has other ingredients that appeal to you. Be careful, however, not to pick a dish that is screamingly high in calories. You don't want to acquire a taste for something that you have to get rid of. Even though you will be modifying the recipe over time to allow the vegetable flavor to come through, it probably isn't a good idea to start liking something a certain way, then find out that it's too high in calories—a potentially good habit gone bad.

If you turn your vegetable course into the main dish, then it certainly can contain more calories than if it were a side dish. Eggplant, large portabella mushrooms, and peppers lend themselves to becoming main dishes. Using cheese as your protein instead of meat, chicken, or fish allows for a meal that is quite filling, and yet easily within caloric limits.

Do you like chili? Make a vegetable chili. You can put all kinds of cut up vegetables in it, and it will still taste just like chili.

How about the spaghetti squash you learned about earlier? You can have a whole plate of it with marinara sauce—quite filling, but also very low in calories. Two cups of spaghetti squash has less than one hundred calories. Covered with marinara sauce, it essentially tastes like marinara sauce, thanks to its bland flavor.

I think I've made my point. You should try to have whichever new vegetable you've decided to acquire a taste for at least two or three times per week for at least six weeks. Remember, you cannot acquire a taste for something unless you repeat the experience often.

It is important that you be patient with yourself, but at the same time, try to be persistent. The world is full of successful people who failed many times before they found success in their endeavors. Don't give up trying to like vegetables. It will make the job of healthy eating so much easier!

Chapter Nineteen

June 2006

When Victor appeared at Cheryl's doorstep the following evening, she was so flustered. Teresa had been keeping her company, and she definitely hadn't been expecting this. She just stared at him in shock, having temporarily reverted back to her old mute self.

Her handsome Al Pacino look-alike was there at her house, unbidden. *Oh my gosh, I must look an absolute wreck*, she thought.

Victor stood there awkwardly with a bunch of fresh flowers in his hand. "Uh, would it be all right if I came in?"

"Oh! I'm so sorry," she blurted out. "Please, please come in." She stood aside and let Victor enter.

"Here." He thrust the flowers toward her. "I, umm, wanted to, uh, bring you something, but, umm, I, uh, didn't know what was appropriate." His fumbling actually made Cheryl feel a bit better about her own awkwardness.

"They're beautiful. Please, make yourself comfortable in the living room. I'll ... ah ... I'll just find a vase to put these in," Cheryl said, happy to escape to the kitchen with something purposeful to do.

Before Cheryl could head to the kitchen, Teresa jumped in. "Can I get you anything to drink?" she asked him. "There's beer, wine, soda ... whatever you want."

"I'll have a beer, thanks."

"Lite or regular?"

"Regular."

Teresa followed Cheryl into the kitchen.

"Gosh, Teresa, what am I going to do? I look just dreadful. I'm so embarrassed. What do I say? Should I change clothes? I'm a nervous wreck."

"Cheryl, just relax and be yourself."

"Easy for you to say." Cheryl really was in turmoil. She wanted to go change her clothes and put on some makeup. But at the same time, it would be so obvious; she knew it really wasn't the right thing to do. After arranging the flowers in the vase, she went into the laundry room off the kitchen, found a small mirror, and tried to somehow improve her appearance. She fluffed her hair, pinched her cheeks, smoothed her eyebrows, and tried to wipe off the faint smudge of black under each of her lower set of lashes. That done, she picked up the flowers and walked into the living room, hiding behind the vase.

"I'm so sorry about your mother, Cheryl," Victor said. "Had I known, I would've come sooner."

"Thank you for coming, Victor. If it weren't for all my friends, I don't know how I would have gotten through these past few weeks."

"Do you think you'll be coming back to the studio anytime soon?"

"I don't think so. I'm not ready to go out just yet. I'm going back to work next week, though. They called and pleaded with me. Sounds like they're in desperate straits, so I agreed to try. I think I'll just wait and see how it goes."

"Can I get you another beer?" Teresa observed the almost finished bottle.

"Please." Victor took the last swig and handed the empty bottle to her.

When Cheryl and he were alone, Victor began. "You know, we miss you at the dance classes—no, I should correct that. I miss you, both at the dance classes and the parties."

"I miss being there ..." She began to reprocess what he said. Her heart began to pound. "I miss you too," she said, ever so quietly.

"You do?" Victor said even more quietly, then cleared his throat. "You do?" he said more loudly.

Cheryl nodded her head up and down, slowly at first.

She saw Victor smile and mimic her nod very slowly.

She smiled back and purposely began nodding more vigorously.

He smiled more broadly, then got up, walked over to her, sat down next to her, and took her hand. He looked directly into her eyes and held her hand. "Did you really miss me?" His uncertainty was almost amusing. Didn't he already know, after all this time?

"Yes, I really missed you, Victor." Neither of them said another thing. They just stared into each other's eyes, trying to read each other's thoughts.

Cheryl heard the front door slam; Teresa must have let herself out. She felt grateful. She wanted this moment to last. Cheryl and Victor just sat looking at each other for quite some time. Eventually, Victor took Cheryl in his arms and just held her. Cheryl didn't know why, but as soon as he did that, she just burst into tears. He held her tighter, just letting her cry. When she'd stopped crying, he just sat with her, holding her hand in companionable silence.

"I don't know why that happened," Cheryl finally said, apologetically.

"You don't need a reason," Victor answered reassuringly. He got up, collected the now somewhat warm beer that Teresa had left on the table, and sat down next to Cheryl. He put his arm across her shoulders and encouraged her to rest her head on his shoulder. He drank his beer as she rested with her head on his shoulder, enjoying the silence and the nearness of him.

Finally, it was getting late, and Victor reluctantly excused himself. He told Cheryl he had an early start in the morning. Cheryl walked him to the door.

"Thank you for coming." As she said that, she kissed him on the cheek.

He kissed her on the forehead and said, "The pleasure was all mine."

He turned and left. She closed the door and turned to lean back against it, her hands still clutching the knob behind her. She was happy and sad, all at the same time. "Oh Mama, if only you could see me now," she croaked, half singing and half whispering the lyrics from an old Barbra Streisand tune.

Victor really, really liked her. She wanted to run into Charlotte's bedroom and share the good news with her. She knew it would make her mother happy. Walking over to the mantel, she took down a portrait of her mother and held it to her breast. She talked to her mom, telling her how she felt and how she wished Charlotte could be there to share her feelings. She told Charlotte how much she loved her and missed her. Cheryl felt very sad, but for the first time in a long time, she didn't burst into tears. She could be unhappy without crying. She walked around the house, looking at and touching things that belonged to her mom. Picking up a bottle of Charlotte's favorite perfume, she pulled out the stopper and let the scent pass under her nose. It was comforting. It was almost as though her mother were still in the room. Tomorrow, when she went to the hospital, she would tell Charlotte all about Victor.

She finally crawled into bed and fell asleep while thinking of Victor. She was hopeful; it felt good.

The next morning, Cheryl was up bright and early. She couldn't wait to get to the hospital to share the good news about Victor with her mother. But before she was able to get out the door, the doorbell rang.

It was a detective. He flashed his badge. "Are you Mrs. Morris?" he asked, somewhat tentatively, glancing down at some notes. From the look of surprise on his face, he was looking for Charlotte, not Cheryl.

"You must mean my mother. I'm afraid she's in the hospital. I was on my way there now."

"Could I speak to you, then, for just a few minutes?"

"What about?"

"Could we step inside the house for a moment? I would prefer not to talk on the street."

Cheryl became nervous. She had no idea what the problem was, but detectives were not usually bearers of good tidings.

"Could you please sit down?" he requested.

She sat on the edge of the couch, looking ready to flee at a moment's notice.

"I think, Miss Morris ... it is Miss Morris, isn't it?"

Cheryl nodded. "Yes—go on!"

"I believe I have what you might consider good news. The man who struck and killed your sister has been caught. He was taken into custody several months ago on an unrelated case. When we ran his DNA against outstanding cases, it matched the DNA from your sister's case. We have subsequently matched both his fingerprints and his DNA to the car that you had identified so many years ago, recovered near the highway. He will be prosecuted."

Cheryl burst into tears. The detective was caught off guard; obviously expecting a more positive reaction. Cheryl was happy. But she was sad that her mother wasn't awake to hear the news. She tried to explain the situation to the detective, but she was so overwhelmed by emotion that her words came out in disjointed, sobbing gasps. Finally, after she calmed down a little, he got the gist of what she was saying.

"You can tell your mother, Miss Morris. She'll hear you. I'm sure of it."

The detective got up to leave. Cheryl stood up and extended her hand. "Thank you, Mr. ... uh ..."

"Mahoney—Detective James Mahoney."

"Thank you, Detective. Let me see you to the door." She started walking toward the door, then stopped and turned to face the detective. "You never told me this man's name or anything about him."

"No, I didn't. His name is Curtis Cummings. He only lived a few blocks from here back then; he lived with his mother and worked for the telephone company. There were no red flags, nothing to connect him to your sister. He didn't have a police record and hadn't worked anywhere that required fingerprints, so he managed to get away with it."

"I don't recognize the name. Do you have a photograph?"

Detective Mahoney pulled out a photograph and showed it to her.

Cheryl looked at it carefully. It depicted no one she recognized. The man in the picture didn't look evil. In fact, he looked pretty much like an average joe. He had brown eyes and brown hair. He wasn't handsome, but actually, almost pleasant looking. He didn't have beady eyes or any other telltale signs that he could kill someone with abandon and just take off as though he hadn't a care in the world. That made it even creepier.

Cheryl turned away and headed for the door again. The detective followed.

"Thanks again, Detective Mahoney. I'll be sure to tell my mother."

She closed the door after him, not yet ready to go off to the hospital. She wanted to digest everything. Life was really funny—not ha-ha funny, weird funny. Neither she nor Charlotte had spoken Joy's name aloud in years until a few months ago, and now this.

If only her mother would wake up, Cheryl would be the happiest girl in the world. She thought of Victor and how good she felt when she was with him. It made her smile.

Once at the hospital, Cheryl eagerly waited for the nurse to leave the room; she wanted a little privacy. Finally alone with her mother, she babbled on for over an hour. She told Charlotte all about Victor, leaving nothing out. Then she repeated what the detective had said. She was holding Charlotte's hand, and Cheryl could have sworn she felt movement. But maybe that was just wishful thinking. Her mom was still resting very peacefully, no signs of wakefulness.

Charlotte was still on a respirator, but the hospital staff had performed a tracheotomy last week, so she no longer had the tube coming out of her mouth. At least it made her look more comfortable.

Cheryl spent the rest of the morning with her mom, but left the hospital at lunchtime. She had errands to run, especially if she were going to start work again next week.

Cheryl called Teresa on her cell phone on the way out of the hospital to share all her good news. Teresa had been expecting a call first thing in the morning; she wanted the scoop on Victor and had expected to get all the nitty-gritty details. She was shocked to hear Cheryl's other news.

"Did you tell your mom?" Teresa wanted to know.

"Of course. I had to tell her first, didn't I?"

"Right. I can be a little dense sometimes. Sorry. So, when are you going to see Victor again?"

"I don't know. He said he would call me."

"Let me be the first to know." She paused slightly. "I'm such an idiot. I'll take seconds."

Cheryl smiled. Teresa was such a good friend. "You'll know soon enough," she responded. "I'll call you tonight."

Cheryl headed home, feeling happier than she had in a long time. Her mom might be in a coma, but somehow, Charlotte was still there for her.

Chapter Twenty

June 2006

The next afternoon, Victor called Cheryl. She had gotten home from the hospital moments before. "Hello, Cheryl?" he asked when Cheryl picked up the phone.

"Yes ... who is this?" Cheryl didn't recognize Victor's voice. She had never heard it over a telephone before.

"It's me ... Victor," he said very nervously.

"Oh!" Cheryl's heart picked up speed. She tried desperately to find the right thing to say. After a split second that seemed like hours, she finally said, "Your voice sounds so much older on the phone. I didn't recognize you. Thanks so much for coming over last night. You ... you made me feel better."

"I'm glad, Cheryl," he said. "That's kind of why I was calling. I have a day off tomorrow, and I was wondering if it would be all right if I came over again. Perhaps there are some things I could help you with."

Cheryl had been praying that Victor would call. She was delighted that he had done it right away—no cat-and-mouse games. That was good.

"I'd really like nothing more, Victor. Thank you."

"What's a good time?"

"How about sometime after lunch?" Cheryl wanted to have time to go to the hospital, get the house in order, and wash her hair. She wanted to look her best.

"Perfect, I'll be there at two."

For the rest of the day, Cheryl ran around straightening and cleaning. Halfway through the job, the vacuum cleaner broke down. *Well, Victor said he wanted to help.* She wondered how handy he was. When she went into the kitchen around dinnertime, one of the bulbs blew. She was kind of happy about that; it gave Victor something else to do. His visit might be less awkward if they had things to do together. As she threw a Lean Cuisine in the oven for dinner, she thought that maybe she could make dinner for the two of them. That way, he'd stay longer.

But did she have anything in the house to make? She looked in the freezer. She had some pounded chicken breast. She could make that with the special low-cal sauce recipe that Dr. Lang had given her. Some veggies and a salad would round out the meal. Then she realized that maybe it wouldn't be enough for Victor.

She could give him a second piece of chicken and make a potato for him in the microwave. She could probably borrow one from Mrs. Curtis; Cheryl was sure her neighbor wouldn't mind.

The next day, after she'd gotten back home from the hospital, she knocked on Mollie's back door. It opened immediately. Mollie smiled the moment Cheryl saw her, gave her a great big hug, and asked, "Now, to what do I owe this visit, young lady?"

"I wanted to know if I could borrow a potato," Cheryl said a little sheepishly.

"My dear, you don't have to borrow a potato—you can have a potato. But are you sure that you don't want more than one?"

"I'm quite sure," Cheryl replied firmly.

"Can I ask what you're going to do with just one potato?" Mollie asked, absolutely filled with curiosity.

Cheryl began to blush.

"You're blushing, Cheryl Morris! I do believe there must be a man involved. Am I right? I bet it's that nice young man, Victor. Yes?"

Cheryl blushed some more and nodded.

"That's wonderful, darling! Come over here and let me give you another great big hug." And she did. "And if ever you need anything, anything at all, I'm always here for you. You know that, Cheryl, don't you?" Mollie handed her the potato.

"Yes, Mrs. Curtis, I do know that. Thanks for the potato, and really ... thanks for everything."

Cheryl returned home to make herself some lunch and begin dinner preparations. She wanted to make the sauce for the chicken ahead of time. It was so easy, but tasted so good that she wanted Victor to think it was far more complicated than it was.

She made her sandwich first. She used low-carb bread that had only forty calories per slice and over two grams of fiber. It was made by Wonder Bread and cheaper than the Weight Watchers and Atkins brand. *No wonder Atkins went bankrupt!* She spread the Smart Beat imitation mayonnaise on each slice, piled on lettuce and tomato, added some thinly sliced turkey (bunching it up to give it more flavor), and then ground some fresh pepper on top. The result was a wonderfully hearty-looking sandwich for less than 300 calories, leaving room for one of her frozen fruit pops—no sugar added—for dessert.

She sat down and enjoyed her lunch. Her mind wondered over the ingredients of the sandwich again, and an image of a warehouse full of the food she hadn't eaten popped into her head. For whatever reason, she hadn't remembered that notion until now. She suddenly had a vision of a building with boxes and barrels of Kentucky Fried Chicken bulging out of its windows. She smiled and wondered if their stock price had gone down since she'd stopped buying it.

Checking her watch, she saw it was one o'clock. She still had an hour before Victor arrived. After lunch, she quickly made her sauce.

She took one tablespoon of Smart Beat imitation mayonnaise, one tablespoon of dark mustard, juice from a small wedge of a lemon, and about a quarter to a half a packet of Splenda, then mixed it and put it in the fridge so that it would be ready to heat up in the microwave for twenty seconds. The entire concoction only had about fifteen calories. It tasted like a fancy honey-mustard sauce. Victor would think that she was a good cook. Little did he know!

Cheryl had another interesting thought. She realized that she was making one of her better fancier dinners, and it was healthy and low cal. She smiled at what Dr. Lang had said—that forming good habits was key. She had never learned to cook before, so she only knew how to cook mostly healthy things. If she had been cooking for years, she probably would have ended up making some fancy high-fat meal. She rechecked that everything was ready to be put together for dinner, then made a mad dash around the house. Lastly, she freshened her makeup, determined to make up for the cosmetic disaster of Victor's last visit. The doorbell rang. It was two o'clock on the button.

Victor looked really sexy to her. He was wearing a mock turtleneck with a cashmere sports jacket, but had dressed the outfit down with jeans and loafers. An unruly cowlick fell forward over his forehead, but added character to his face. The best part was his smile. When he smiled, his eyes crinkled and twinkled. He was smiling when she opened the door.

This time, Cheryl ushered him right into the house without staring at him on the doorstep, as she had the day before yesterday.

"Can I get you something to drink?" she asked a little nervously. *Why does he do that to me? I've talked to him thousands of times—no need to be so nervous.*

"No, thanks. I just had lunch."

As they walked into the living room, Victor almost tripped over the vacuum cleaner, which Cheryl left there on purpose.

"Oh, sorry! I left it there because it broke down on me a few hours ago, and since you offered to help, I thought maybe we could start with trying to fix that thing."

Victor smiled. "I'll be happy to try." He shed his jacket and laid it over the back of one of the large living-room chairs, then dropped to his hands and knees to see what needed to be done.

"Do you have any screwdrivers?" Victor asked.

"In the shed in the backyard."

They both went back there, and Victor rooted around for the tools he might need. It took a little while to find the right size screwdriver, but after that, Victor made the repair look simple. It seemed that the belt had come off, and it just needed to be put back on and tightened. It took Victor a little while to figure out how to take it apart. But once he finally got it apart, he explained to her what he was doing as he was fixing it.

"You made that look so simple," Cheryl remarked.

"It was simple," Victor retorted.

"Not to me, it wasn't."

Victor smiled. "So what else did you have in mind for Mr. Fixit here?"

"Well, conveniently, the kitchen fixture just blew. I have new bulbs, but the light fixture is a little complicated."

That task proved to be a little more complicated than they had first thought because of the way the fixture had been put together. When they finally got the cover down, it was apparent that most of it needed a good washing.

After finishing those chores, they sat in the living room—Victor with a beer, Cheryl with a Diet Pepsi. (Yes, she had finally realized that she now enjoyed Diet Pepsi.) The conversation just flowed between them both. Once they had gotten over their mutual shyness, they realized how much they had in common. They liked the same music, books, and movies. Neither one of them was very interested in sports. Cheryl actually loved to dance more than Victor, but that was only because his mother had made him do it all the time. In truth, he did enjoy it, because it made up for his otherwise awkward demeanor.

They shared their pasts and some of their trials and tribulations. On one occasion, Cheryl began to cry because of a story she was telling about her mother. Victor just handed her his handkerchief, put his arm around her, and let her bawl. He didn't get upset or try to cheer her up. He just let her stop crying on her own time. And when she did, they were both comfortable with the silence.

"God, where has the time gone? It's already dinnertime. You're staying for dinner?" Cheryl said it more like a statement then a question.

"I never turn down a free meal, especially when a pretty girl is making it."

They went into the kitchen together.

Victor insisted on making the salad, rooting around in the cupboard to find the ingredients to make his own salad dressing from scratch.

Cheryl knew that she had to make the chicken just before they were ready to sit down, so she had saved that for last. She had put the nonstick frying pan, greased with cooking spray, on the stovetop. She then put the potato on a dinner plate in the microwave for a total of four minutes, turning it over after two. Then she pulled it out, cut it open on top lengthwise and crosswise, and squeezed it at the bottom to open it up a little more. She seasoned it with a little butter, salt, pepper, parsley, and a slice of cheddar cheese; Victor didn't need to worry about calories. She put the potato aside to be reheated right before she took the chicken out of the pan.

She took the other dinner plate and put the frozen whole green beans on it. She seasoned them by spraying them first with a little butter-flavored cooking spray, so the seasonings would stick. Then she added salt, pepper, and onion powder. She put them in the microwave for three minutes, took them out, tossed them, and put them aside. During this time, Victor was still preparing the salad and the dressing. Before he had completed his task, though, Cheryl had lit the gas burner under the frying pan.

By the time Victor was finished preparing the salad, the pan was hot enough for the already seasoned and pounded chicken breasts.

"Where do you keep the plates and flatware?" Victor asked. "I'll set the table while you finish dinner."

While the chicken breasts sizzled, Cheryl finished Victor's potato by putting it in the microwave for another minute. She then put the beans in for another minute and a half, tasting one to make sure it was cooked to her satisfaction. She flipped over the chicken breasts and then retrieved the sauce from the fridge and heated it for twenty seconds. She took half the string beans and added them to the dinner plate that held Victor's potato, then sprinkled them with thinly sliced almonds. By that time, the chicken breasts were finished cooking. She gave herself one piece and Victor two, then coated them with her honey-mustard sauce. The total cooking time was under twenty minutes, and everything had been cooked just right. And on top of that, cleanup would be a cinch—so few dishes.

During the entire time they were preparing dinner together, the conversation had continued to run smoothly—which Cheryl had found truly remarkable.

She was equally impressed and pleasantly surprised at her own newly developed cooking skills, having learned the importance of timing. Victor seemed impressed as well.

"This is delicious," he finally said after a few minutes of companionable chewing.

"This salad dressing is great as well. Where'd you learn to cook?"

"Hey, I'm a single guy. Gotta learn sometime."

"I suppose, but most people would just pour it out of a store-bought bottle."

"I like to be creative. That way, I can make it the way I like it."

"Hmmm. That's funny."

"What's funny?"

"That's kind of what my doctor's been telling me about learning how to cook."

"You do cook. This chicken is really good; you'll have to give me the recipe."

Cheryl smiled. *He thinks I'm a good cook—that's a laugh. Hopefully, I can keep my secret a while.* "Thank you," she said demurely.

It was so incredible how comfortable she felt having him around. Cheryl was beginning to feel as if she had known him her entire life. She was pretty sure this wasn't going to end as previous relationships had: in disaster.

The time continued to pass by so quickly; Cheryl couldn't believe it. Dinner had come and gone very successfully, and now it was getting late and time to part. They stood at the door, saying an awkward good night. To kiss or not to kiss? Finally, Victor made a move. He put his arms around Cheryl, pulled her close, and very gently and very tentatively kissed her on the lips. Cheryl returned the kiss eagerly. He pulled his head back and looked in her eyes, gauging her willingness to kiss him again. This next kiss was a little harder, and a little more urgent. He hesitantly flicked his tongue into her mouth; she flicked back. He began to explore her mouth; she opened hers wider. Cheryl's legs became very weak … and then weaker still as she felt his reaction to her. Victor pulled away. He was breathing fast, but no faster than Cheryl. He wasn't smiling, but his eyes still twinkled. Cheryl thought she was going to pass out.

"I, um, think I better go," Victor mumbled.

Cheryl nodded. "Good night," she said. "You'll call me tomorrow?"

"You can bet on it! Oh, and Cheryl, thanks again for dinner. It was really good. I didn't know you were such a good cook."

"You're welcome. You certainly know your way around the kitchen. You make a mean salad."

"Good night … I'll call you tomorrow." With that, he backed out the door, almost falling off the top step.

Cheryl couldn't help but smile. She had begun to notice that as graceful and suave as Victor was on the dance floor, he was actually a bit of a klutz. She thought it was kind of endearing. She was beginning to learn that Victor was, in a way, two different people. At the studio, he was a talented man about town, but in most other environments, he was shy, reserved, and a bit awkward—someone who needed looking after. Cheryl really liked him. In fact, if she were truly honest with herself, she was falling in love with him. She prayed that he felt the same.

While Cheryl was waiting for Victor to arrive, she remembered the warehouse, picturing it full of Kentucky Fried Chicken. Can imagining a warehouse full of uneaten food help you to achieve your goals?

WHAT HAPPENED TO THAT WAREHOUSE?
By
Nikki Lang, MD

In the beginning of this book, we had discussed creating a warehouse full of foods that you wouldn't eat for a year. At that time, we put sixty-one cases of juice or soda on the shelves to represent the two cans a day that had been given up. We also put five five-pound bags of sugar and one two-pound bag of sugar to represent the two teaspoons of sugar in two cups of coffee a day.

Let's make some other calculations for fun to give you an idea of what that uneaten food represents. Let's suppose that, although you haven't given up Italian hoagies yet, you've made some modifications. First of all, you leave off the cheese and the mayonnaise (or the oil). Since you've got lettuce, tomatoes, onions, and hot peppers, you've decided the sandwich is moist enough without them. You also request that your deli dig out the roll before they make the sandwich. Let's also assume that you eat a hoagie three times per week. Italian cheeses are usually sliced more thinly, so let's assume there's twenty slices per pound, and four slices per hoagie. Let's also assume two tablespoons of mayonnaise per hoagie. Lastly, let's guesstimate that the amount of bread pulled out from the middle of the roll represents about one and a half slices of bread. (An Italian hoagie roll has 400 calories. Italian bread is 70 calories per slice. So 1 1/2 slices would represent about 112 calories or just over a quarter of the roll.)

One and a half slices of bread 3 times per week for 52 weeks equals 234 slices of bread. Divide this number by the amount of slices in a loaf (20), and we have almost 12 loaves of bread in our warehouse.

Four slices of cheese 3 times per week times 52 weeks equals 624 slices. If we are assuming that a pound of cheese holds 20 slices, then 624 slices divided by 20 gives us just over 31 pounds of cheese that we can put into our warehouse. Two tablespoons of mayonnaise 3 times per week for 52 weeks equals 312 tablespoons of mayonnaise. There are 16 tablespoons to a cup, and a standard jar of mayonnaise holds 2 cups (16 ounces). If we divide 312 by 32, we get almost ten (9.75) jars of mayonnaise in our warehouse.

Now think about what we've just discussed. Just by digging out the hoagie roll, leaving off the cheese, and skipping the mayonnaise, our warehouse of uneaten food now contains

31 pounds of cheese
12 loaves of bread
10 jars of mayonnaise

Mind-boggling, isn't it? Let's look at another possibility. Let's say you found my recipe for pizza made on a high-fiber tortilla with sauce, mushrooms, spinach, and peppers. You've been eating that with a salad instead of regular pizza, when you would otherwise indulge in two slices. Since my recipe with the salad is equal to one regular slice of pizza, then you are not eating that second slice of pizza. Since you do this three times a week, then you are saving three slices of pizza per week. Three slices of uneaten pizza for 52 weeks comes to 156 slices. Dividing by 8 (slices in a pizza), you realize that your warehouse currently holds nineteen and a half pizzas!

When you have created some new habits that allow you to eliminate certain foods from your diet, it can be fun to perform this exercise. With a mental picture of that warehouse full of food, you can begin to understand how important those small changes are. I have chosen the above examples to point out that we don't necessarily need to give up everything in order to make a big difference.

That hoagie we discussed above will still have an awful lot of calories. But if you were to divide it in half or in thirds—depending, of course, on the size of the hoagie—you could have a third at 10:30, a third at 1:30, and a third at 4:30. You might be thinking that a third or a half of a hoagie would never satisfy you. But remember, if your habit was to not eat breakfast and then eat that hoagie at lunchtime, when you're starving, it wouldn't have been as satisfying to eat just a half or a third. This time, however, you'll have already eaten breakfast, and you won't be all that hungry by 10:30, or at 1:00 or 1:30.

This exercise of creating a warehouse can be very helpful in improving your determination to succeed. Discuss it with your friends, and have fun with it.

Chapter Twenty-One

July to September 2006

Two weeks after starting an antidepressant, Cheryl had her follow-up appointment with Dr. Lang. She figured that the medicine must be doing something, because she really was sleeping better and not worrying so much during the afternoons. Victor probably reckoned into the equation as well. But if she was really honest with herself, she had started to sleep a little better even before Victor had arrived on the scene.

What Cheryl was really interested in, though, was her blood work. Some time after her last office visit, she had realized that she had forgotten to take her sugar medication ever since her mother had become comatose. So when the blood was drawn, she had been off her medication for several weeks. She certainly hadn't planned it that way, but now she was hoping that if it all was good, she wouldn't have to take the medication anymore.

Dr. Lang entered the exam room, wearing her usual jeans and Docksiders. Today, though, she was wearing a bright yellow Gap shirt instead of white, black, or blue, and her hair was pulled back in a ponytail. That was unusual, but it was certainly cheerful.

"I have your lab tests back, and Cheryl, they were all good. The cholesterol is still a little off, but again, I think we can address that at a later date. But your sugar and hemoglobin A1C are perfect. You've done a great job. How are you feeling otherwise? Are you sleeping any better?"

"Doctor, I have a confession to make. In all the confusion following my mother's heart attack, I forgot to take my diabetes medication. Since my blood work was so good without it, do you think maybe I could stop taking it altogether?"

"Probably, though before I commit to that, I'd like to check a fasting insulin level just to make certain. So, are you sleeping better?"

"Oh, yes, much better … and my days are going better as well."

"I see that your weight is still 191, the same as it was the last visit. Under the circumstances, that's very good. When are you going back to work?"

"I'm starting back on Monday. To tell you the truth, I'm looking forward to it. It'll keep me busy."

"So maybe you could begin to get back on track?"

"That's my plan. I'm not really up to dancing just yet, but hopefully fairly soon."

"Sounds good. Why don't you try to come back some morning next week before work to get that fasting insulin level, just so we can confirm that you really don't need to take the medication?"

"I will, Doctor. I promise."

"How about I see you in one month?"

"Okay … see you then."

Cheryl was very happy that she might not need to take the diabetes medication anymore. But she understood Dr. Lang's concern, and she would still take it if Dr. Lang deemed it necessary. She would definitely get it checked out.

Cheryl slowly got back into a routine. Work was a bit difficult at first, because everyone was visibly uncomfortable, not knowing what to say. Eventually, though, everything finally went back to normal. Tina continued to order lunch for her when she forgot to bring something, but she was, in fact, remembering more often to pack three small meals. She ate the fourth meal on the way home on the bus.

Victor came around regularly. He helped her around the house, and they sat and talked and rented movies. All in all, they had found comfort in each other's company. They were still a bit shy about kissing or making out; Cheryl felt an additional warmth and closeness toward Victor when she sensed that Victor was being very careful not to take advantage of her vulnerability.

After several weeks, though, he had begun asking Cheryl to come back for her dance lessons. "Why don't you come for a lesson tomorrow?" Victor asked as he was leaving.

"I'm really not ready yet," she answered. "You know, when I started working, everyone was so ill at ease. No one seemed to know how to act around me, and I'm just not ready for a whole dance class of people acting uncomfortable. I don't want to start crying in front of everyone. Can you understand that?".

"Sure I can. I'd just really like to see you get out and enjoy yourself more. You know, I have an idea, if you don't mind. Since you don't want to come to a class, what if we went out, just the two of us, for dinner and dancing—at Brasil's, maybe? The music is great. They have salsa dancing, and we could have a really nice dinner. How about I take you out on Saturday? After all, I owe you a bunch of dinners. You've made dinner for me so many times."

Cheryl was weakening. *Maybe it's time I got out of the house a little …* "Come on, it'll be fun. Pretty please," he pleaded. She finally nodded her consent. He threw his arms around her and gave her a loud smack on the lips, making her laugh.

Cheryl's spirits really were picking up. Last week, she had gotten her test results in the mail. Her insulin levels were good. She could truly stop taking the medication. When she found out, she immediately went to the hospital to tell her mom. When she'd arrived, she was very pleasantly surprised. In spite of Charlotte's coma, they had been able to wean her off the respirator. Her color wasn't as good as it had been on the respirator, but she actually looked well. Cheryl had renewed hope that her mother might get better.

Cheryl was definitely getting back on track with her eating program. She even started getting off the bus a few blocks away from her regular stop and walking briskly the rest of the way to work. In addition, she had decided to move her bedroom back upstairs. She'd thought that the added necessity of running up and down the stairs would put a little more exercise into her life, since she wasn't dancing. She even managed a few nights of salsa practice with the weight vest on. She was amazed at how much endurance she had lost over a number of weeks. If she was going dancing on Saturday, she had to brush up. She was pleased that she had agreed to go and hadn't realized how much she was looking forward to it until she began practicing again.

Oh, my, she thought. *Do I have anything to wear?* She didn't think so. She wondered if Teresa was free to help her shop for something.

Teresa wasn't home and didn't answer her cell. Cheryl left a voice mail that she desperately needed Teresa's help.

Teresa finally got back to Cheryl; she had turned off her cell phone. It had been one of those rare nights when she'd gotten to see Michael. Yes, miraculously, they were still an item.

"So, what's the crisis? I thought things were going swimmingly well with Victor."

"Oh, they are, but he asked me out to Brasil's Saturday night, and I have absolutely nothing to wear. You're so much better at picking out clothes than I am. You always manage to pick out just the right thing." With her initial weight gain, Cheryl had lost her flair for choosing her own clothes. She'd thought that everything made her look fat.

"Flattery will get you everywhere!" Teresa responded, pleased by Cheryl's compliment. "When can you go?"

"How about tomorrow after work? Can you escape the store?"

"Sure—I'm not working tomorrow night. I'll meet you at your office, and we'll go from there."

"You're a lifesaver!" Cheryl exclaimed and hung up.

Cheryl must have tried on fifty different outfits at four different stores before they found the right one. Finally, they accidentally encountered the perfect casual dress, right when another woman walked out of a fitting room wearing it. It was a somewhat flashy print—not something that either of them would've picked up off a rack. But it had such a nice cut, and the material flowed so well. It didn't look at all cheesy, despite how it appeared on the hanger. Teresa and Cheryl gazed at the woman examining herself in the three-way mirror, then looked at each other. They couldn't find Cheryl's size on the rack, so Teresa hovered around the other customer until the customer had given it up to the lady manning the dressing room.

Teresa arrived at Cheryl's stall triumphantly, dress in hand. Cheryl put it on, and from the minute she zipped it up, there was no doubt that it was the right one.

"And I know just the perfect pair of shoes for it!" Teresa exclaimed. "Let's go back by the store, so I can show them to you." They did, and as usual, Teresa was right on. The shoes looked great with it. "Do you have a purse to match?" Teresa asked.

"I do, actually," Cheryl responded. "And thank goodness I do. The prices you charge in this store could make me go bankrupt!"

"You only get what you pay for," Teresa retorted. "They are, after all, well-made designer shoes and handbags."

"I know, I know … it just makes me feel better to complain about it. Thanks a million, Teresa. I couldn't have done it without you, as usual." She gave her friend a hug and started to go out the door.

"Hey, hold on. I've got my car here today; I can give you a ride. Just give me a second. It's at the lot near Second and Lombard." Teresa gathered up her stuff and checked with her employee to make certain everything was under control.

On the way home, Teresa grilled Cheryl about Victor.

"So, what's Victor like in bed?"

"Teresa!" Cheryl practically screeched her name. "You're so … so … crude!"

"Does that mean he's not any good?" Teresa asked, laughing.

"No, it doesn't! I mean … I don't know." Cheryl was getting flustered.

"You're not serious. You mean … you two haven't done the deed yet?" Teresa really had a hard time believing her. "What in heaven's name have you been doing with all the time you've spent together?"

"We watch movies, talk a lot about things, cook, and listen to music. You know, stuff like that."

Teresa was skeptical.

"Geesh, is he gay or something?"

Cheryl remembered some of their kisses and Victor's reaction. "No, I'm pretty sure he isn't. It's just not the right time yet. You know, it's been an awfully long time since I've been with anyone, and I'm just not ready to jump in the sack."

Teresa discarded her teasing tone. "Well, don't wait too long, or he might disappear."

"In all honesty, Teresa, I don't think so. Victor is really someone special. We're getting to know each other, and we like each other. I think when the right time comes, we'll know it."

"If that's what makes you happy. You sure aren't me, though. I'd have been all over him by now."

"Well, thank goodness you don't find him that attractive. I might've never gotten a chance with him."

"I doubt that, Cheryl. He only had eyes for you, right from the beginning. I know you didn't see it, but everyone else did."

"You keep telling me that, but I find it so hard to believe."

"Believe it! Anyway, here we are, back home safe and sound from yet another epic shopping spree. You'll have to let me know how Saturday night goes."

"You'll be the first to know. Well … maybe the second. Somehow, telling my mom first always makes me feel better. You know, Teresa, as crazy as it sounds, I really believe she hears me. Once in a while, I even think she's responding to me. Maybe I'm being foolishly optimistic, but recently, I've gotten the feeling that she's waking up."

Teresa certainly wasn't about to put a damper on Cheryl's optimism, and Cheryl could tell Teresa was choosing her next words carefully. "Maybe she is, Cheryl. Let's keep our fingers crossed."

Cheryl went to bed that night feeling particularly positive about the future. As she drifted off to sleep, a barely discernible smile appeared on her face as she thought of her upcoming date with Victor.

Chapter Twenty-Two

September 2006

Cheryl was ready for her date a little early. She kept peeking out her window, looking for Victor. She'd been brimming with anticipation and excitement all day; she kept dropping things and forgetting stuff in her discombobulation. She really couldn't understand why she was so nervous. She had spent many very comfortable evenings with Victor, so what was so different about tonight?

Again, she looked out the window. Victor was nowhere to be seen. She looked at her watch. He was a few minutes late. She became a bit apprehensive. Mulling over her feelings, she reviewed the past couple of weeks, thinking about how comfortable she was with Victor. She realized that this was actually their very first date. No wonder she was worried—she was venturing out on a date for the first time in ages. Would the date run as smoothly as their evenings at home? A dab of adrenaline coursed through her body. Her heart sped up a tad, and her palms began to sweat. She took a sniff of her underarms. They were okay. She made another mirror check. Her face was flushed. The doorbell rang. Thank goodness!

Cheryl opened the door. Victor stood on the doorstep—at least, she was pretty sure it was Victor. She saw two legs and half a body supporting a large bunch of flowers—gladiolas, one of her favorites. She couldn't believe he had remembered. A voice filtered through the flowers. "I know I'm late—sorry. Traffic was a little heavier than usual. Something big must be happening at the Spectrum. Am I forgiven?" For insurance, he thrust the flowers forward.

"They're beautiful!" she exclaimed. "You remembered. You're so sweet." She took the flowers, leaned over them, stood up on her tiptoes, and kissed him on the cheek. "Let me just shove them in a vase so we won't be late."

She ran into the kitchen, found an old vase, put in some water, and plopped the flowers in. She grabbed her coat and then Victor's arm, and they were out the door. Victor opened the car door for her and helped her into his Honda Accord. She realized that she hadn't known what kind of car he drove. Victor was never lucky enough to find a parking space anywhere near her house—a phenomenon not unusual in South Philly. She was relieved that he didn't own a bachelor show-off car. The interior was immaculate. She wondered whether he had cleaned it up for their date. The thought gave her pleasure.

As they approached Chestnut Street, Victor spotted a parking spot. After the car came to a complete stop, Victor turned off the ignition and started out the door. He was stopped abruptly by his seat belt, which he had forgotten to release. Cheryl stifled a giggle.

Victor smoothed his cowlick back into place, released the belt, and rushed around to Cheryl's door, taking her hand as she emerged from the vehicle. She enjoyed the chivalrous gesture. The restaurant was all she had hoped for—warm, comfortable, and not too sophisticated. Some of the "in" restaurants today were too cold for her—all that granite and stainless steel combined with a cool palette. They might be considered fab by the yuppie crowds, but to her, they were very unwelcoming and intimidating.

Their table was small and intimate. They ordered drinks; Victor ordered a vodka and tonic. Cheryl made a mental note. She had no vodka in the house. Cheryl ordered a Virgin Mary. She chose two appetizers for dinner—one to have when Victor had his appetizer and one to have as dinner. Victor ordered a bottle of wine and two glasses. Cheryl let him pour her a small portion of wine. In doing so, he knocked over the water glass. Cheryl jumped up, and fortunately, no damage was done. Victor blushed and couldn't stop apologizing. Cheryl had to keep from smiling at the sight of his reddened face. Victor was so sweet.

They finished their dinner. Cheryl did end up drinking about a half of a glass of wine. She really wasn't crazy about the taste of alcohol, but she did feel relaxed.

The music had begun. Cheryl didn't want to dance until others were doing so. Apparently, most of the dancing didn't occur until much later. Finally, one or two couples filtered onto the dance floor. Victor very gallantly got up and bowed in front of Cheryl, extending his hand. "May I have the pleasure of this dance?"

Cheryl chuckled at such a formal gesture but put her hand in his and allowed herself to be led to the dance floor.

Her lack of practice made for slow going at first, but after about five minutes, they were right in step with each other. Cheryl wanted to sit out the next couple of dances. She was out of breath. In spite of the few practice sessions at home, she was not back in shape. She was surprised at how quickly her endurance had diminished.

Once they were really warmed up, though, they got better and better. At one point, they were the only ones on the floor, and several people applauded when they were finished. The praise made Cheryl's night. She actually indulged herself in another half glass of wine. She felt slightly inebriated—not to mention exhausted from all the dancing. She suggested they go home, and Victor agreed.

Once the pair arrived back at Cheryl's doorstep, the same ineptness plagued them both. Cheryl, feeling flush with wine and the excitement from all the dancing, suggested Victor come in. He was most agreeable. She asked if she could get him anything to drink, and he asked for another glass of wine. She had some left over from a previous night's dinner. She poured a glass of wine for Victor and a caffeine-free Diet Pepsi for herself. When she brought the drinks into the living room, Victor motioned for her to sit next to him.

"It was an absolutely wonderful evening," Cheryl remarked. "I'm so glad you suggested it."

"It was wonderful," Victor said softly. You're wonderful." And with that, Victor took her into his arms and kissed her with such passion that Cheryl felt faint. He was no longer able to hold back. He began kissing her all over—her forehead, cheeks, ears, and neck. Chills shot up and down her spine. Victor really turned her on. She couldn't remember when she had last felt such desire.

Cheryl unlocked their lips and pushed him back with her hands on his shoulders. "Let's go upstairs," she whispered.

Victor looked into her eyes; he was breathing hard. "Are you sure? Are you really sure?"

"Yes, I'm really sure," Cheryl responded. Now was the right time.

Once in the bedroom, Cheryl refused to turn on any lights. She was still ashamed of her body—still convinced she was fat. They undressed on opposite sides of the bed, their backs to each other, and slipped between the covers as quickly as they could. Victor pulled her to him, again covering her with small, light kisses. What followed seemed like the most natural thing in the world, as if it had always been meant to be.

"Why are you crying?" Victor inquired afterward with great concern.

Cheryl opened her eyes and responded tentatively, "I think … because I'm so happy?"

Victor looked into her glistening eyes, then surprised Cheryl with tears of his own. Cheryl looked at his brimming eyes with wonderment, and then with joy.

And suddenly, the two of them started laughing together.

"A fine pair we make," Cheryl said, half crying, and half laughing.

"We do make a fine pair," Victor answered, wiping the tears from his face.

"Why do you suppose you're crying?" she asked.

"I suppose it's just happiness and pent-up emotions," he answered. "But you know what? It's okay. In fact, it's good. I'm not ashamed of crying. There's nothing wrong with feeling." Victor's tone held a touch of defiance.

"Hey, buddy, I'm all with you. I agree," Cheryl concurred.

"And now that we've done the dirty deed," Victor continued, ripping off the covers, "Let me finally get a look at my fair maiden."

"Nooooo!" Cheryl grabbed the covers back up, resisting vehemently.

"Please," Victor pleaded. "I really do love your body. At least let me admire it. You're so beautiful. What's wrong with wanting to look at something so beautiful?" He looked like a kid eager to unwrap his Christmas present.

Cheryl held tightly to the covers and shook her head vigorously.

"Can I at least turn on the lights?" he asked.

Cheryl was horrified. "No!" she said quite firmly.

He looked crestfallen, but he didn't push it. Instead, he gently licked the tears he had found at the corners of her eyes and then kissed each lid. He took her head in both hands, and when she opened her eyes, she found him gazing at her face with such love that Cheryl's stomach lurched, and her heart sped up. She hugged him even tighter, if that were possible. She just couldn't get close enough.

They got very little sleep that night, reveling in the love they had both found. Fortunately, Victor had had the foresight to take Sunday off, so they were able to sleep late.

Morning could've been uncomfortable, but it wasn't. Victor hopped out of bed first and into the shower. By the time Cheryl had come downstairs, he was busy making breakfast. After last night, he was incredibly hungry, and now he was making one of his famous Spanish omelets. He had cut and sectioned a grapefruit for her, brewed coffee, and made her sit down while he served breakfast. She declined the toast.

Cheryl really couldn't believe her good fortune. Victor was everything she wished he could be, and more. Under the table, she crossed her fingers.

"This omelet is really good," Cheryl said.

"I make a mean cheese omelet as well, but I thought it might just be too many calories for you."

Now, how did I manage to be so lucky? He cooks and is thoughtful too!

While cleaning up the kitchen, Victor began singing a bit off-key. Cheryl chimed in, her voice no better than Victor's. They tried to outdo each other by singing further off key, ultimately erupting into laughter.

"Anything you can sing, I can sing better!" she sang, just as awfully as she had sung everything else.

"No, you can't!" he sang back, catching her reference to that *Annie Get Your Gun* tune despite her lousy pitch.

"Yes, I can. Yes, I can. Yes, I can!" she sang back.

"No, you can't," he said, poking her in the ribs. She poked back. He deliberately began tickling her. She tried to tickle back but charged off into the living room instead. He ran after her, caught up with her, threw her on the couch, and began tickling her unmercifully. She laughed so hard, tears were rolling down her cheeks. She could hardly breathe.

"Please stop," she said in a choked voice. He stopped and instead starting kissing her again.

"Let's go back to bed," Victor suggested.

"I'd love nothing more, baby, but I really have to get some chores done, and I really have to get to the hospital."

"You're right … I should be going. I have an awful lot to do as well." He got up and took Cheryl's hand to help her up. Once she was up, he pulled her toward him. He kissed her very lightly on the forehead and on the cheeks. "I'm going to miss you."

"Me too. I mean, I'm going to miss you too." They hugged each other in silence for a few more seconds.

Victor let go reluctantly and headed for the door. "I'll call you tomorrow."

Cheryl watched him through the window until he was no longer in sight. *He makes me happy*, she thought. *I've never felt this way about a man before.*

Cheryl finally felt ready to tackle some of the paperwork that had been hanging over her. Her mother used to take care of all the bills, but for obvious reasons, it had become Cheryl's responsibility.

Cheryl worked hard through the rest of the day, pausing from time to time to daydream. She'd made up her mind that it was time to resume dancing lessons. Victor might like her body the way it was, but she didn't. She still wanted to lose the rest of the weight and resolved to work a little harder.

Chapter Twenty-Three

September to October 2006

The next day, while the two women ate lunch in the conference room, Tina looked at Cheryl and remarked, "You look different. I can't quite put my finger on it, but there's definitely something different about you today."

Cheryl continued chewing and said nothing, but unfortunately, her face reddened ever so slightly. Tina started to laugh and said, "Well, I'll be. You and Victor have finally done it. Haven't you?"

Cheryl's face turned scarlet, and she put a finger to her lips to shush Tina. "Come on, Tina! You're not supposed to talk about things like that. Pipe down, or Dr. Weiner will hear you."

"What, you think he's a virgin?"

"Shush! I told you stop talking like that."

Tina started chanting in a singsong voice, "Cheryl's gotten la-id. Cheryl's finally done it."

Janie rushed in. "What's all the commotion?"

"See? I told you to be quiet," Cheryl scolded.

"So, what's goin' on?" Janie wanted to know.

This time, Tina spoke very quietly, "Cheryl's not a born-again virgin anymore."

"Really? Victor?" Janie inquired.

"Is nothing sacred around here?" Cheryl queried.

"Aw, c'mon, Cheryl. What's he like? You can tell us!"

"I can't, and I won't … at least not yet. It's too personal and too private. I'm not used to this."

As Cheryl left the room, she heard Tina say, "She'll give it up sooner or later."

The rest of the day, Cheryl endured dozens of little remarks and innuendos. Cheryl alternately blushed and smiled, even giggling occasionally. She found that, oddly enough, she enjoyed being teased by the girls. In a way, it made her feel more a part of the group.

Cheryl couldn't believe how busy she was over the next number of weeks. She started dancing again twice a week. Victor came over a couple of nights during the week, and they usually went out on Friday, Saturday, or Sunday, depending on his schedule at the studio. Between shopping, cleaning, cooking, dancing, and visits to the convalescent home—they had transferred Charlotte from the hospital, since she was no longer on a respirator—she barely had time to think. Making time to eat healthily was, without question, difficult. She really did have to consciously set aside time in her schedule. She was beginning to understand how important it was to prioritize her weight-loss goals.

Cheryl had forgotten her follow-up appointment with Dr. Lang. She got a notice in the mail telling her that if she failed to show up for a second missed appointment, she'd owe a twenty-five-dollar fee. She felt awful; she wasn't usually that irresponsible. When she had received the notice, she suddenly recalled that not only had she missed her appointment, but she had also failed to take her anti-depressant pills. She guessed that she didn't need them anymore. She was sleeping just fine. She'd have to call, apologize, and reschedule an appointment.

When Latisha put Cheryl on the scale, she was surprised. Cheryl now weighed 171 pounds. "That's really great, Cheryl," Latisha remarked. "Most people don't have the patience to do this right."

"I guess I'm not most people," Cheryl responded. As she followed Latisha to an exam room, she thought about that. She wouldn't have made such an assertive comment a year ago. Her self-esteem must really be improving.

While she was waiting for Dr. Lang, her mind wandered over all the changes that had taken place during the past year and a half or so. She had become a dancer—a good one—and a cook. She was admittedly not a fabulous cook, but she was a cook nonetheless. She'd had to assume many of her mother's responsibilities and no longer had her to depend on, and Victor was now a permanent part of her life. She had lost sixty-four pounds, and not only was she keeping it off, but she was losing even more. She was amazed that her eating habits really had changed. She liked the food she ate now. She no longer craved Kentucky Fried Chicken or french fries. The most astounding surprise regarding food had come this last week, however.

She had decided, one day, to treat herself to a Snickers bar after all this time, but she hadn't been able to finish it. It wasn't that she didn't like it, she did. But after a few bites, she had had enough. It was almost too sweet and too rich. She wrapped it up and saved it. It was still sitting at the bottom of her purse. Now, that was flabbergasting! Dr. Lang was so right. Patience and acquired taste really were the crucial elements to the process.

She thought about that time at Carol's house, when the girls had conspired to get her drinking diet soda all night. None of this might have happened if they hadn't done that, or if Teresa hadn't gone with her for dance lessons. Without those lessons, Cheryl might still be a slug—maybe a somewhat thinner slug, but a slug nonetheless. So much of her life had changed.

By the time Dr. Lang walked into the exam room, Cheryl wanted to hug her. "Dr. Lang, would it be inappropriate if I gave you a hug?"

"Absolutely not. I like hugs."

Cheryl hugged her and thanked her. "I know I'm not done yet, Dr. Lang, but I'm sure I will get there. You were very hard on me in the beginning, and I simply couldn't understand what it was all about. Now, I understand that it really is about an attitude more than anything."

"Yes, Cheryl—attitude, patience, and knowledge. Thanks for that hug. How are you doing otherwise?"

"Really great. I stopped taking the antidepressant. I just didn't need it anymore."

"That's fine; it was just to help you get over a hurdle without falling down. How's the healthy eating coming?"

"I'm doing well. The habits are there. I am doing the Atkins thing a couple of times a week, which seems to be helping, and I also started walking more. I get off the bus way before my stop, and sometimes after work, I do a fast walk back to the same stop."

"Great! Then there's just one more chapter of my book that I'd like to give you. It's called 'Fine-Tuning Your Calories.' It's a bit complicated in that there's a fair amount of math, but it will help you determine how many calories you should be eating to maintain your ideal weight. When you do get to your ideal weight, you should remeasure your body fat to make a more accurate calculation."

"You don't need to make another appointment unless you want to, though I would like to recheck your blood work in about six months. I want to keep an eye on your cholesterol."

"Will do ... and Doc, thanks again."

"You're more than welcome. You have no idea how much pleasure it gives me to see you succeed."

On the bus going home, Cheryl glanced at the chapter she had been handed. It was a bit confusing. She decided to save it for a morning read, when she was more alert and could concentrate better.

Victor was coming over that evening. She was looking forward to it, as usual. She popped a Lean Cuisine in the oven; she didn't feel like cooking tonight. She was cleaning up the kitchen when Victor appeared. While she stood at the sink, Victor slipped his arms around her from behind and kissed the nape of her neck. It sent chills down her spine and made her knees weak.

"How's the most beautiful dental assistant in the world?"

She turned around and kissed him on the nose. "Just fine. Can I get you anything to drink?"

"Sure—I'd love a beer." Cheryl complied, and they both went into the living room. Cheryl turned on the TV and checked the guide to see what was on. Victor took the remote from her and turned it off.

"Before we get involved in any programs, I'd like to ask you something."

"Ask away."

"Do you have any plans for Thanksgiving?"

Cheryl had deliberately not thought about it. With her mother in the convalescent home and only distant family members left, she wasn't sure what she was going to do.

"No, I don't have any plans at all. I haven't even thought about it. Why?"

"I'd like you to join our family for Thanksgiving dinner. Not that my family is all that big, but I'd really like you to come. I've already checked with my mom, and she's all for it."

Cheryl beamed and kissed him. "Of course! I'd love to meet your family."

That settled, on went the TV, and they discussed which program to watch. They nixed a movie for something shorter, so they could be in bed early. Victor slept over these days and left for work in the morning. He didn't have to leave as early as Cheryl, so she had given him a key to the house. They were thinking of moving in together, but Cheryl was unable to make any decisions like that while her mother remained in coma. Besides, they had plenty of time.

**Cheryl admitted that making time for a healthy lifestyle is difficult.
Can you find that time?**

ON MAKING TIME
By
Nikki Lang, MD

When I discuss diet with my patients for the first time, I am constantly amazed at the depth and breadth of the emotional reactions that accompany the conversation. Frequently, patients become tearful. They don't always cry, but I can see the tears welling in their eyes. Often, they get angry with me. They've reconciled their obesity with their self-image, and I shouldn't upset the apple cart. Or they're sure that I couldn't possibly understand their particular situation. Sometimes, they just get annoyed, and you can almost hear their thoughts: *Here we go again.* Occasionally, they listen with great enthusiasm, but tired skepticism is more likely. They've tried so many times to diet and failed. They already know it's not going to work; their eyes just sort of glaze over.

Although this chapter should probably be in the beginning of the book and not toward the end, I've chosen this spot because I wanted you to understand the process first. Why? Because of the reactions mentioned above.

As I previously stated, changing habits is not easy. Most people prefer not to disturb the status quo. It's easier to keep things the way they are and rationalize the impossibility of change. It's much easier to give up and make excuses as to why we can't do what we know we need to do.

I have, throughout this book, emphasized that eating habits involve changing many habits, not all directly related to eating. I've hinted at one of the most important changes, but have not come out and discussed it directly. I've talked about spending a little more time at the grocery store each month, along with a little more time packaging and preparing your meals the night before, so you can take them with you to work the next day. I've also discussed taking that extra time to study local restaurant menus. The thing that I have not discussed directly is just how much of your very valuable time that is required to make these changes.

While you have been reading this book, I have no doubt that one of the recurring thoughts running through your head was something like this: *That's all very well for her to say, but my schedule is so difficult. She has no clue how impossible it would be for me to do all of this.*

I agree that we live in a very demanding world, and time is precious. So let's just discuss how you might make enough time to accomplish many of the changes we have already discussed.

We cannot discuss making time for something, without discussing the need for setting priorities. Simply put, you have to decide what matters most to you. Stated another way, you have to decide what must be done, what might get done, and what can be left for another time.

For example, going to work takes top priority in most people's lives. They have to make a living. Keeping yourself clean and appropriately dressed falls into a top priority as well. After all, you want to keep your job and not offend co-workers, friends, and family. Eating is a top priority. You need fuel to function. Sleeping is also a top priority, though the amount of hours of sleep required will also vary quite a bit. So clearly, the majority of any given day is taken up by things we have to do, and the few hours left to our discretion have to be doled out very carefully. How we ration out those precious hours will determine our success or failure at any given task.

Finding the extra five or ten minutes in the morning to eat breakfast might mean giving up five or ten minutes of sleep time, or it could mean giving up relaxation time on the weekend to teach your four-year-old to dress his or herself, so you can eat breakfast every morning instead of dressing your child. Collecting menus from local eateries might mean giving up some downtime chatting with co-workers on your lunch break. Preparing meals for the next day the night before might mean giving up some sleep or possibly giving up watching a TV show. We work very hard and deserve rest and relaxation. Nobody will deny that, but you need to decide which activities are the more important ones as each day goes by.

My job, if I am going to be successful in getting you to adhere to this program, is to convince you that losing weight matters. It's not the top priority, certainly, but it ranks sufficiently up there on the priority totem pole to warrant effort.

Your health is probably one of the most important aspects of your life. If you remain healthy, you can continue to do your job, be there for your family, and—most importantly—feel good. When you're not healthy, it costs you money for medications. It costs you time away from work—and therefore even more money. Not being healthy can make you unhappy or depressed. Obesity is just about the number-one health risk in this country. It is a major contributing factor to high blood pressure, diabetes, and heart disease.

Not being overweight increases your chances for a longer, healthier, and happy life. I realize that you probably already know these things. So I guess the next question is, why not make your health a priority? Why does everyone and everything take priority over you? I can't answer that question for you. But I have a suggestion to make. Perhaps if you put yourself first, maybe you might begin to like yourself a bit more.

So now we see that making positive changes requires setting priorities by putting yourself toward the head of the line. What does that mean in day-to-day terms?

How often do we do something solely because we don't want to upset someone or we want people to like us? Whether we are at work or in a social situation, this frequently happens to most of us. How do we let this happen, and more importantly, what can we do about it? Just as important, how will it give us those extra hours we need to make those changes?

Ever have a friend call you to go out to go to a movie, or have a drink, or whatever, just as you were about to wash your hair, or do the laundry, or some other household chore? You're mentally all set to do whatever you had planned, and somehow you're convinced to go out and put off what you had planned until the next time. You really didn't want to go, but he or she twisted your arm. Why?

Did you tell them what you had planned for the evening, then allow them to convince you otherwise? That's mistake number one. If you want to put yourself first, before your friends or family, and yet not offend them, recognize that it is important not to give a specific explanation as to why you can't do something. He or she does not want to play second fiddle to hair washing. The only thing you need to do is allow your friend to save face. You can simply say, "I'd really like to—you know how much I enjoy your company. But I can't go; I already have plans." In the beginning, it may be difficult for you, but the more often you say no without giving an explanation, the more it will be accepted, as long as you do spend time with this person now and then. If you always say no, then, of course, he or she will stop calling. But if you always say no, then maybe that's a good thing, as you really didn't want to spend any extra time with them in the first place. Time is really such a valuable commodity—think twice before giving it away so easily.

Suppose you're at work, and a colleague repeatedly asks you to do small jobs for him or her. And because you're such a nice guy or gal, you always do it. At times, you really should be saying, "I'd really like to help you out, but this time I've got to say no. I'm just too overwhelmed with my own work—sorry."

You can see how putting yourself before others can garner some additional time for yourself.

What about the workaholic? If your job requires ten- and twelve-hour days, then maybe you have to ask yourself which aspects of your job are more important than your health. Try to work out some compromises with yourself to squeeze in a little extra time.

Sometimes, I find that the more intelligent a person is, the quicker he or she is to come up with some amazing rationalizations as to why something is impossible. Why not use that intelligence to figure out a solution?

One of the suggestions I've made before is to pretend that you are your own client. Pose the dilemma you are having to yourself, then come up with solutions to the problem. What would you tell a friend struggling through this same dilemma? We are often much better at solving other people's problems than our own. Reduce your emotional involvement, and find a solution.

Hopefully, I've convinced you that you need to make yourself a priority in your life. If I have, then most of what we've been talking about will become a little easier to do.

Now that we've broken down psychological barriers, I'd like to discuss practical ways to find time in your day. Ideally, we should all be able to afford an efficiency expert that could follow us for a week and then tell us how we could save time. Unfortunately, none of us can afford that, so we'll just have to take a peek at some common ways that people waste time.

Being over fifty, I find that I waste the most time looking for things. Where'd I put the keys? Where are my glasses? Where'd I put the sponge? Where's my checkbook? I could have sworn I left the umbrella by the door. I do, however, do this less and less.

I get so angry with myself when I waste time needlessly, so I make extra effort to always put things back in the same place I found them. Granted, I don't always succeed, but I keep trying and have made some progress. Spending those few extra seconds or minutes putting something back in its original spot sure does save a lot of time in the long run.

Let's talk about grocery shopping, a subject that's a bit more on target here. Everyone does his or her grocery shopping in a different way. Some people go once a month and spend several hours, some go once a week, and others go every other day to pick up a few items at a time. Which is the best way? Well, there really is no best way, but there is always a more efficient way.

If you stop off at the local food mart or grocery store every other day (because you don't have time to do a big shop), how long does it really take? Well, if you're driving, you have to stop at the store, then spend a few minutes parking and walking. You then have to enter the store and find what you want (ten minutes?). Then you have to wait in line. Perhaps you're lucky, and the express line only has one or two other people in it (another ten minutes?). Then you have to take your groceries out, put them in the car, and find your way back toward home (five minutes or much more, depending on where you live). So you just spent around a half hour (if you're lucky) on a "quick stop," and you do this three or even four times a week? That means you spend anywhere from one and a half to two hours a week shopping. And you say you don't have time to do a big shop? How often do we really examine how inefficiently we spend our time?

What if you did a major shop once a month? (Needless to say, you'd have to have a large freezer.) That usually takes, all in all, about three hours. But then, once every ten days or so, you'd have to stop for milk, or lettuce, or other perishable items, which could take half an hour each stop. This method adds up to about four and a half hours a month, or just over one hour per week. You'll save anywhere from two to four hours per month.

What if you rarely stop at the market, but tend to eat out a lot or grab something on the way home? I don't need to tell you that eating out takes much more time than eating in. Even ordering takeout will add up to more time than it would take to make something at home—and cost more too. You have to go out of your way to stop at the eatery, order your food, wait until it is prepared, pay for it, and then find your way home. Ordering takeout may be less of a hassle, but it isn't necessarily faster.

Lists can be real time savers. If you write down everything you need to get before you go out, you can save the time you would have spent going after those forgotten items.

I think by now you get the picture. If you give your schedule some thought and rearrange your priorities, you can find the time you need. As we stated before, little changes add up. You can do most of the things you would like to do, especially if they're important enough to you. You just really need to want something badly enough to make it happen.

If reading this chapter has upset you or made you angry, then you may want to gain more insight into those feelings. Perhaps a coach, a minister, or a therapist might be helpful in achieving that goal. Losing weight may not be simple for you; you might be deeply and emotionally invested in eating.

Although on the surface, what I have said in this chapter makes an awful lot of common sense, I realize from my many years of experience as a family practitioner that this information can offend people, despite my good intentions. Please don't be offended. Rather, understand that your emotional investment is the problem and seek help. It will be the first step to a healthier—and, hopefully, happier—life.

Chapter Twenty-Four

November 2006

Cheryl had stopped at the pharmacy on the way to Teresa's shoe store to pick up a couple of sundries. As she passed by the gym on Fifth Street between Bainbridge and South, she noticed a sign in the window: Determine Your Body Fat for Free. Although she had no intention of utilizing their facilities and realized it was just a come-on, she decided, *What the hell.* She went in and kind of wandered around a little until she saw someone she could talk to.

"I saw your sign in the window. I'd like to measure my body fat."

"Sure, no problem," responded the trainer, who wore tight Lycra pants and a top that accented his bulging muscles. "Follow me." He took Cheryl into a small room and put her on a scale—one more elaborate than the one in Dr. Lang's office. After asking her for her age and height, the trainer plugged in some numbers, noted she was female, and came up with 33 percent. Cheryl was pleased. She had been at 37 percent.

"Now you know, of course, that you should only have 27 percent body fat, tops. We have a program here to get that body fat off. We have an introductory free session, and after that, it's only thirty dollars per month. Training sessions are extra—"

Cheryl interrupted, "I'm in a hurry right now. I was supposed to meet someone a few minutes ago." To be polite, she added, "But if you could give me some literature, I'll be back in touch." She still had no intention of joining a gym, but at least she knew what her body fat content was. Maybe she would sit down and do those calculations this weekend.

She tossed the gym brochure in the nearest city trash can after she rounded the corner. She was definitely pleased. Maybe by the time she reached her goal weight of 145, her body fat would be even less.

Teresa and Cheryl had their dance lesson tonight, but Cheryl had finished work a little early, so she thought she'd stop in the store and see if there was anything new in stock she might be interested in. Teresa was with a customer, so she wandered around looking at shoes, most of which she had seen before. Nothing new.

"So, what's up?" Teresa asked when she was free.

"Nothing too much, but Victor asked me to have Thanksgiving dinner with his family."

"Did he, now? Sounds promising—taking you home to meet the family. Not bad. Michael hasn't made any offers like that, but of course he has to go with the team. He doesn't really get to go home for Thanksgiving. But then again, you'd think I'd get to meet his family at some point."

"Where do they live?" Cheryl asked.

"In Phoenixville."

"Well, that's not so far away ... but I bet with his schedule, he rarely gets a chance to go home."

"That's true, but his parents always go to the games when they're playing in Philly. He could make some sort of arrangement after the game, couldn't he? I don't know what to think about it."

"Maybe he will. He probably just isn't quite ready for that."

"But we've been dating longer than you have," Teresa said, whining slightly.

"I know, but you have to admit it's been sort of a long-distance relationship. Granted, Victor and I got a later start, but we've seen a ton more of each other than you and Michael have. Try to be patient, Teresa. If there's anything I've learned in the past couple of years, it's that patience really is a virtue and does pay off in the end."

"Yeah, I guess so."

"And for goodness' sake, don't push him. You know how badly that works out."

"I know," Teresa said somewhat dejectedly. "I do know better than to push, but I really care about him, and I'd really like a signal that he cares for me as well."

"How can he not? You're devastatingly beautiful, and since he doesn't dance, he doesn't know that you're not perfect." Cheryl poked her friend in the rib and laughed, just to make sure Teresa understood that she was just teasing her. "Come on—if we keep jabbering like this, we're going to be late for our lesson."

Class was fun as usual, and contrary to what Cheryl had said earlier, Teresa was becoming a very good dancer. She was very much in demand at the studio parties.

Thanksgiving was almost upon them, and Cheryl was getting a little nervous. What would Victor's family think of her? Would they accept her? And again, what to wear continued to plague her to no end. Since she kept losing weight, nothing ever fit right. She loved the dress she'd bought for their first date, but it was already too loose and didn't lay right. She really wanted to wear it and didn't want to spend the money for another outfit. *If only I could sew, I could fix it*, she thought. But that was never going to happen. Even in high school, when she had taken a class in home economics, it was obvious that sewing was never going to be one of her hobbies.

Suddenly, she remembered that the dry-cleaning store around the corner from work had seamstresses. She could get it fixed there. Why hadn't she ever thought of that before? In fact, why not go through her closet, pick out her favorite things, and take them all there to see what was reasonable to get fixed? Her red dress from New Year's last year had hung in her closet almost an entire year untouched.

Cheryl was excited about the prospect of increasing her wardrobe without spending a fortune. Oh, she knew it wouldn't be cheap, but still, alterations were a lot more economical than buying a new wardrobe. And besides, she really liked a lot of the things she had. A huge amount of time and care had been expended finding those garments in the first place. She wasn't ready to discard them just yet.

*   *   *

Cheryl twirled around in front of the mirror with her newly tailored dress. Almost nineteen months had passed since she embarked on her new weight-loss journey. She was down to 167 pounds and looking good. The alterations had been the right decision. The dress was perfect; the busy print even looked festive and appropriate with its orange and black accents. She pulled her coat out of the closet. It wasn't actually a coat; it was more like a cape. That had been an ideal purchase, as she could wear it at any size. She ran into the kitchen to get a bottle of wine to bring and rummaged around for an appropriate bottle bag to put it in.

Victor would be at her house any minute. She checked her makeup and hair one more time. Satisfied, she relaxed and waited. Victor rang the bell, punctual as usual. He started to open the door with his own key, but Cheryl had gotten there first.

Victor whistled at her. "You look beautiful. Isn't that the dress you wore when we went to Brasil's?" His memory always amazed her. "But you look even better than you did then, and that's saying something. What's different?"

"About twenty pounds and a good seamstress." Cheryl turned all the way around and stepped back for Victor to admire.

"Come here." He stepped forward, pulled her into his arms, and kissed her.

Cheryl pushed him back. "Hey, buster, be careful of the makeup. It took me hours."

"Let's go upstairs for a quickie," Victor suggested.

Cheryl chuckled. It pleased her that he found her so appealing. "We can't. We're going to be late."

"Then what am I going to do about him?" he asked, pointing to his nether regions.

"Oh, poor baby. I guess you'll just have to figure out something else," she said as she grabbed her coat and bottle of wine, purposely brushing by him as she headed out the door.

"That's playing dirty," Victor moaned.

"No … I think what *you* suggested would be considered playing dirty," Cheryl said with a wicked smile.

Cheryl was overwhelmed when they arrived at Victor's mother's home. It was far grander than she had expected and not far from the studio, in a very posh section of town—one of those older, stately town homes. Apparently, the dance studio business was fairly lucrative. Cheryl was immediately intimidated by her surroundings. She hoped she wasn't gawking. But the high ceilings, carved wood-working, and moldings were beautiful. The marble entryway was exquisite, as was the staircase leading to the second floor.

Mrs. DePalma greeted Cheryl very warmly. "Cheryl, I'm so glad you could come. You've made Victor very happy, and anyone who makes my son happy is very, very welcome in my home."

Cheryl started to extend her hand out in formal greeting, but Mrs. DePalma wasn't having any of that. She gave Cheryl a big hug and then put her arm around Cheryl's shoulder. She led Cheryl into the living room, where the rest of the family had been waiting in anticipation.

"Come with me, Cheryl. You must meet the rest of the family. This is Maria, Victor's sister, and Gianni Palermo, her husband. That's Gianni Jr. sitting over there … impolitely playing with his computer game." Mrs. DePalma said that last bit loudly, clearly trying to get his attention. He didn't look up or acknowledge her presence. "And this is Angelina, Maria's youngest."

Angelina looked about five or six. She had been playing with her doll on the floor. But she very carefully stood up and extended her petite hand to Cheryl. "I'm very pleased to meet you," she said gravely.

"I'm very pleased to meet you as well."

"Are you going to dance for us? Victor says you're a great dancer," the little girl said.

"I, uh, don't think so … not tonight. But, uh, thanks for asking me," Cheryl answered, caught off guard by the child's ingenuousness.

"And last, but not least," Mrs. DePalma continued, "I'd like you to meet my brother, Bruno—Bruno Sabitini. He's visiting from Florida. His kids all live down there."

"A pleasure," Bruno said as he took her hand in both of his, bowed, and kissed the back of it. "You are a very beautiful woman. My nephew has very good taste."

"Be careful, Cheryl. He's quite the ladies' man," Mrs. DePalma warned. "He's broken many a heart in his lifetime."

Cheryl laughed. Now she knew where Victor had picked up some of his charm. "Don't worry, Mrs. DePalma. I'll be careful."

"Don't be so formal. Please, call me Anita. Now, can I get you a drink?"

"A Diet Pepsi would be great, thank you."

"Oh, but you must have a glass of wine. We've just gotten the most wonderful case of wine from Argentina. You've got to try some. It is Thanksgiving, after all."

She took Cheryl by the hand and led her to the bar. Bruno slipped behind the bar and poured her a glass of wine from the already opened bottle. Cheryl took a small sip and nodded. "It's good." She still wasn't crazy about wine, but admittedly it was starting to taste somewhat better to her.

They chatted for another half hour or so before Anita announced that dinner was ready. Maria got up first and walked over to Gianni Jr. After she had removed the Game Boy from his clutches, she took his hand and led him into the dining room. Angelina followed with her father. Victor escorted Cheryl, pulled out her chair, and settled her in. Bruno gallantly interlocked his arm with his sister's and said, "Shall we?" then glided alongside her until he reached her seat. He pulled out her chair and mockingly made her wait until he had dusted off some nonexistent crumbs. Then, with a flourish of his arm, he suggested that her chair was now suitable for placing her delicate bum upon. He made Cheryl laugh. He apparently had had a few more drinks earlier and was in a particularly jovial mood.

With everyone seated, dinner began. They all joined hands and bowed their heads for a short prayer of thanksgiving. Victor squeezed Cheryl's hand nice and tight. She liked this family. They made her feel welcome.

Cheryl ended up with much too much food on her plate. She ate a little bit of everything—probably more than she was used to, but she marveled that she really couldn't eat any more. Her stomach must have shrunk from eating all those small meals all the time.

While they were waiting for dessert, Mrs. DePalma proposed a toast. "To my brother, for taking the time out for his sister. It is greatly appreciated. Thank you."

"To my sister, for putting up with a licentious old codger like me!" Bruno responded.

"To my mother," Maria added, "for having the most delicious Thanksgiving dinner I think I've ever eaten."

Cheryl put her wine glass in the air. "I second that," she said. She was surprised when she looked at her nearly empty wine glass. She had had almost two whole glasses of wine. No wonder the room felt so warm.

Victor stood up and cleared his throat. Everyone looked at him in anticipation, "To Cheryl, the most beautiful woman I've ever met, both inside and out." Cheryl's face turned scarlet. Then she watched in fascination as Victor moved his chair back even farther, got down on one knee, and thrust forward a small, opened black box that held the most beautiful ring she had ever seen. "Will you marry me?" he asked, his eyes glistening.

Cheryl was absolutely dumbstruck, and her tongue found its old home at the roof of her mouth. Tears of happiness welled up in her eyes while she nodded vigorously up and down. She threw her arms around Victor and finally said, "Yes, yes, yes. I love you so much. You make me the happiest woman on the planet."

He unraveled himself from Cheryl's arms and placed the ring on her finger. It was just a little big; she had lost weight since he had ordered the ring. "I'll sort that out with the jeweler later," he whispered. As he slipped the ring on her finger, everyone applauded, and one by one they came around to Cheryl, gave her a big hug, and welcomed her to their family. She couldn't stop crying, she was so happy. The only other thing that she could've possibly wished for was the presence of her mother.

"So when should we have the wedding?" Anita asked.

"Hold on, Mom; give her a chance to breathe. She just found out," Victor interceded.

"Well, Cheryl, any thoughts at all on the subject?"

"I need a little time to think about it. Not too soon. Victor's right—I do need some breathing space. Also, I really want it to be special, and I believe with what little I know about weddings, we'll need some lead time to book and so on," Cheryl responded pensively. She also wanted to give herself time to lose the rest of the weight. She didn't want to look back at her wedding album and see a fat girl. Not that she was really fat anymore, but she wanted to be just right.

"Well, Victor told me you don't have much family left, and your mother is still in the convalescent home, so I'm more than happy to help with the planning. It's been a long time since Maria got married, and boy, oh boy, I do enjoy a good party! So please don't remain a stranger. In fact, Victor, why don't you bring Cheryl around for dinner next week, and we can talk about it?"

Victor looked at Cheryl for her approval. "Is that okay with you?"

"Yes … yes, I'd like that," Cheryl responded.

That night, when Victor and Cheryl crawled into bed together, they made the best love ever. He kept referring to her as the future Mrs. DePalma. Cheryl's shyness had slowly waned; she loved the way Victor worshipped her body. He made her feel beautiful.

Sometimes when she would get out of bed nude in the morning, he would follow her with his eyes and remark about how he loved her butt, or her breasts, or even her nicely rounded belly. How perfect she was. She almost began to strut in his presence, and from time to time, she'd purposely make some explicitly sexual moves, which would never fail to arouse him. She loved teasing him. Mostly she loved how much he wanted her. That aroused her more than anything.

She was so happy.

Chapter Twenty-Five

November 2006 to June 2007

The next day, Victor wanted to take the ring back to the jeweler to get it adjusted. Cheryl wasn't having any of that. It wasn't leaving her finger just yet; she wanted to be able to show it off. It wouldn't be the same, telling everyone how he had proposed without the ring to back it up. She couldn't wait to get to work. She wasn't going to say anything; she would wait till someone noticed.

No one did until lunch. Cheryl, of course, had had the ring covered by latex gloves all morning. Everyone had been so busy when she'd first arrived that there had been no opportunity. At lunch, however, as soon as Tina sat down, she was nearly blinded.

"Oh my gosh, Cheryl! I can't believe you didn't say anything. How could you keep something like that all to yourself? Janie, Darlene, Mary, hurry up! You've got to see this. Cheryl, it's absolutely gorgeous. Give me your hand. Let me see it up close."

Cheryl extended out her left hand for Tina to admire. No sooner had she done so than the other girls came in and started oohing and aahing. Even Cheryl couldn't believe how beautiful the ring was. She couldn't have picked out anything prettier. Three diamonds sat in a row on a white gold setting, with the center diamond slightly larger than the other two. There was no doubt about the quality of the diamonds. They had the most amazing brilliance.

The girls were full of questions. How did he pop the question? Where? When? Cheryl told them everything.

"Really? At his mother's, in front of his whole family?" Tina said rhetorically. "How wonderful."

Dinner at Victor's mom's came almost too fast. Cheryl really hadn't given much thought to the wedding details; she had been so busy. She still felt very intimidated when she walked into the house. She wasn't used to so much wealth.

Victor's mother insisted on being called Anita and continued to make Cheryl feel very welcome. Over dinner, everyone told stories about their respective families. Anita said that she was certain that she would've liked Charlotte and was sorry that she might not ever get to know her. Cheryl learned that, although

Anita's family had been wealthy, it wasn't old wealth. Anita's father and grand-father had made most of their money bootlegging during Prohibition. She had some very colorful stories to tell and held no pretenses; she actually poked fun at her family wealth. She hadn't had that much money when Victor and Maria were growing up. Her family wasn't crazy about Anita's choice of husband and let her know it. That was why she worked so hard teaching dancing. She had already started the dance studio here in Philadelphia by the time her father died, leaving her and her brother his fortune.

She knew that Cheryl had no real family to speak of and told her that she was more than willing to foot the bill for the wedding. After all, Victor was her only son. Besides she would hit Victor's father up for part of it; he owed her. Anita explained that she had let him get away with not paying for Maria's wedding. He was too busy getting fleeced by his second wife, who had recently run off with her aerobics instructor. Anita told Cheryl that she had tried to warn him. "But you know men," she said. "Why he had to get involved with someone fifteen years his junior is beyond me. Men never think with their brains, do they?"

Cheryl giggled. She was very satisfied about her ability to make Victor happy. She had been worried that he wouldn't like her body as much when she lost the rest of the weight. She remembered their conversation when she had asked him to help her with the calculations that Dr. Lang had given her. She had told him that her ideal weight was 145 pounds. He balked immediately, arguing that she would be too thin. When she disagreed, he had protested, "But I so love your butt, and your breasts, and your nice round belly ... you know that. They might disappear."

"Have they disappeared yet?" she responded. And he had to admit, she just seemed to get curvier. She seemed to naturally have a beautifully rounded butt that jutted out ever so nicely, in spite of the fact that it had become a little smaller. The same applied to her breasts, and she did continue to get more of a waistline.

He shook his head. "You're right. You're looking better and better. Don't become too beautiful—I don't want anyone stealing you away!"

Cheryl rolled her eyes. "Well, I promise to stay with you if you would just help me with my calculations."

They reviewed Dr. Lang's chapter called "Fine-Tuning Your Calories" together. Cheryl and Victor figured out that at 33 percent body fat and 145 pounds, she would be carrying around almost 48 pounds of fat. *Wow, that sounds a lot better than seventy-two pounds*, thought Cheryl. In that case, her lean body mass would be ninety-seven pounds. They multiplied that by 12.5 and got 1,212.5 calories. They then determined that she probably averaged about 5 calories per pound per day for exercise because, although she'd been getting a lot of exercise dancing, she literally sat around all day at work. Calculating 5 x 145 determined that she burned 725 calories from daily activity. If she added those two figures together, she could eat around 1,938 calories per day to maintain her ideal weight of 145. If she divided that by 5, each meal could contain 387 calories—probably more than she was eating, but she was still trying to lose weight.

The weeks went by at a very rapid pace. By necessity, Cheryl spent a lot of time with Anita. She really liked Anita and was happy she was going to have a mother-in-law. She had heard all those mother-in-law jokes, but she knew that with Anita, those stories wouldn't be true. They had finally agreed to have the wedding in June. Anita wanted to have it sooner, but Cheryl wanted a little more time. Besides, she'd always wanted a June wedding.

Christmas and New Year's flew by, both celebrated at the DePalma residence. The wedding plans were well under way. Cheryl had decided that if her mother remained in a coma, she was going to sell the house, and she and Victor would buy a house together. Anita suggested that they move into her house, as there was so much room, but Victor and Cheryl both vetoed the idea, deciding instead that they wouldn't mind a house nearby.

The real-estate market had gone bonkers in the past couple of years. Cheryl couldn't believe how much her house was worth. But by the same token, she was shocked by the cost of a tiny house not far from her future mother-in-law. Cheryl and Victor both really wanted to stay in town and start a family really soon, so they hankered after something with a small backyard. They had a fair amount of money to spend between the two of them, but didn't want to become house poor.

Cheryl couldn't believe how quickly time was going by. The invitations had gone out, but she hadn't yet bought a wedding dress—she was waiting until the very last minute. She wanted to lose as much weight as possible before trying on dresses. She'd even started doing additional exercising so that she could lose weight a little faster. Anita was pestering her and pestering her, warning her that she wasn't going to have a wedding dress if she didn't start looking yesterday to find one.

Finally, Cheryl agreed. Now weighing 152 pounds, she figured another four or five pounds wouldn't make that much of a difference in dress size.

Cheryl was spending more time with Anita than any of her friends. She hardly had any time for anything else. She couldn't believe how time-consuming planning a wedding could be. She was also looking for a house and buying a trousseau. Imagine that: she was buying a trousseau and planning a honeymoon! They hadn't yet agreed on a destination. Cheryl wasn't so sure about the Caribbean. She couldn't picture herself in a swimsuit yet.

Victor told Cheryl that he had spoken to his dad on several occasions. Victor had wanted him to come up and meet Cheryl before the big day. His father had said that wasn't possible, but he wouldn't miss the wedding for anything in the world. He made sure to say that he was very happy for his son, but Cheryl could tell Victor was angry. Victor told Cheryl his father never seemed to have time for him. His father was such a bright man. How could he always find time for bimbos, but not his own son?

Cheryl was so grateful to Anita. A fairytale wedding was in the works, and Cheryl knew that none of it would've happened if Anita hadn't done the planning. Cheryl had had a great deal of trouble making decisions, especially when it came to spending someone else's money. But in the end, it was exactly the kind of wedding she wanted for herself, held outdoors at a beautiful old estate. (The grand salon in the house wasn't quite large enough to accommodate the ever-growing guest list, but Cheryl had always wanted to have an outside ceremony anyway. Why else have a June wedding?)

They decided not to have a sit-down meal, opting for a variety of hors d'oeuvres instead. They would be serving all kinds of different foods in different rooms. Several different bars would be open so that people could come and go as they wished, as well as eat when they wanted. Dancing would be in the grand salon. They had hired a very versatile band that could play swing and salsa as well as some jazz.

Through many conversations, Cheryl knew that Victor was getting increasingly upset that his father still hadn't come to Philadelphia. He had promised to come at least a few days before the ceremony. But with just two days to go, no one had heard anything. Cheryl tried to calm Victor down, but when the topic of his father came up, he would get angrier and angrier. Cheryl just tried to avoid the discussion altogether.

Cheryl had found the perfect wedding dress, and amazingly, it had almost fit perfectly right off the rack. Over the last several weeks, she had, at Anita's insistence, sampled all the food that was going to be served. It was amazing. Some of it was absolutely foreign to her tongue, but all of it was incredibly delicious. And although it hadn't been all completely healthy, an awful lot of it met Cheryl's demands.

Both Victor and Cheryl had had the requisite bachelor parties. They were equally as bawdy, but Cheryl's party had become particularly rowdy when Teresa arrived flashing her new engagement ring—Michael had finally proposed. Everyone's happiness escalated, feeding off each other's raucous laughter, and Cheryl had even allowed herself to get drunk. Under the influence, she finally provided the girls with the lascivious details of Victor's prowess in bed. They accused her of exaggerating, but she denied it vigorously. She knew they were all jealous, but she also knew she probably would be just as jealous if one of her friends described what she had. He was a fabulous lover, no question about it.

Cheryl and Victor agreed not to see each other the day before the wedding. They'd spent the previous night together, but Victor was not the best company, because he still hadn't heard from his father, and he was brooding. Cheryl tried to comfort him. She even did something that she had never done before: she seduced him. She actually came downstairs to the living room wearing just a sexy gown on and started to do a striptease of sorts, exposing only one part of her body at a time while moving in a very seductive way. She hummed slow music while she did it.

At first, Victor tried to ignore her, but found he couldn't. He started to smile. "What have I created?" he asked. She didn't answer. She just kept humming and moving in time with her music. She slowly approached him, then wrapped her arms and legs around him. In spite of being fully clothed, he moaned, "You win, baby." He picked her up as he got up. Cheryl marveled that he could actually pick her up. He carried her upstairs and made mad passionate love to her … and then he cried.

She knew what he was thinking: *Where is my father? Doesn't he care about me at all?*

Cheryl held him tight and said nothing—the same courtesy that he had extended to her when she was hurting so. Nothing more was said. They parted in the morning, not to see each other until their wedding.

"I love you," Victor said. "I'm going to miss you."

"I love you too." They rubbed noses. "And I'm going to miss you too," Cheryl said in an almost childlike voice.

They separated reluctantly. Victor struggled with the lock on the door and then nearly tripped on his way out. Cheryl smiled. *God, I love him so much.*

> # Can you calculate how many calories you'll need to consume to maintain your ideal weight?

STEP 8: FINE-TUNING YOUR CALORIES
By
Nikki Lang, MD

After reading some of the previous chapters, especially those on metabolism, you may be asking yourself, *With all the variations in calorie requirements, how can Dr. Lang recommend, across the board, 350-calorie meals for women and 450-calorie meals for men?*

When I started this book, I mentioned that I didn't want to get too technical too early. After much calculation, I determined that the above calorie recommendations are an excellent place to start. Once you begin to get the hang of the process, then perhaps a little fine-tuning will be in order.

There is a reason that 300-350 calories per meal is a good place to start. A fifty-calorie difference in each of the five meals gives you a daily difference of 250 calories. Since most of us are not particularly exacting, it's not unreasonable to expect this kind of variation. When translated into daily calories, this meal guideline gives a daily range of 1,500-2,000 (350 x 5 +/- 250) calories per day for women and 2,000-2,500 (450 x 5 +/- 250) for men. When you do the more exacting calculations, most people who have a weight problem will need to stay in these calorie ranges.

In the beginning, the increased metabolic speed from five small meals a day is going to have the most impact on weight loss. As time goes on, and weight loss occurs, it will become more important to determine a more exact number to maintain your ideal weight. This can be done by more rigorous calculations or simply by trial and error over time. If you are weighing yourself frequently, as I suggested, you will see the weight coming off slowly over time. If that stops happening over a two- to three-week period, and no weight is being lost, then you'll have to shave a few more calories off each of your five meals.

If you are exercising more and building more muscle mass as time goes on, you will be able to eat more calories and still lose weight. You might encounter plateaus, where nothing happens for a while. That's really okay as long as you make sure you don't put weight back on, which is why it is important to weigh yourself regularly.

Your ideal weight really needs to be determined by you. I can give you all sorts of charts that list recommended weights according to size and body build, but they don't always fit everyone. You probably know already what weight you would be happy achieving and maintaining, and that should be your ideal weight goal. Charts cannot take into account the extra weight you might carry in your legs or buttocks, and if you go only by height and bone structure, a chart might put you at a weight that is much too low, causing you to look much too thin and drawn in the face.

I will, however, discuss some guidelines for those of you who have absolutely no idea how much you should weigh. Please skip this part if you already know what your ideal weight should be. I don't want you obsessing over a weight that is unrealistic.

Generally, women should weigh 100 pounds for the first five feet, and then, depending on bone structure, so many pounds for each inch above five feet. Someone with a small frame can multiply each inch above five feet by 5; someone with a medium frame can multiply each inch above five feet by 6.5; and someone with a large frame can multiply each inch by 8. Therefore, an average woman with a small frame who is five foot four inches should weigh about 120 pounds, whereas a woman of the same height who has a large frame should weigh about 132 pounds. Remember, these are only guidelines; they aren't written in stone.

Men, on the other hand, should weigh 106 pounds for the first five feet, and then one additional pound more than a woman for each inch over five feet. So a small-framed man who is five foot ten inches tall should weigh approximately 166 pounds (106 + (10 x 6)), and a large-framed man at the same height should weigh about 196 pounds (106 + (10 x 9)). Also, if you are over forty, it would not be unreasonable to add ten pounds to the above result.

Mathematically determining caloric requirements for maintaining your ideal weight can get a bit more complicated. I will try to explain it as simply as possible, laying out a formula at the end where you can plug in your own numbers. If math really turns you off, just ignore it all and utilize the practical approach discussed above. These calculations are mentioned only for those who have a need to know or would feel more comfortable with more specific guidelines.

One of the difficulties in determining appropriate caloric intake is knowing what your body-fat percentage will be when you get there. Even if you have your body fat measured today, that does not mean it will be the same later (quite frankly, I hope not) when you arrive at your ideal weight. So for the purpose of completing our calculations, I am going to make certain assumptions. When you do arrive at or near your ideal weight, you can certainly have your body fat remeasured. Hopefully, if you then continue to exercise and build muscle, your caloric requirement will increase, and you will be able to consume more calories per day while still maintaining your ideal weight.

A top normal body-fat percentage for a woman over thirty is 27 percent, and for a man over thirty, it's 23 percent. Most obese women that I have measured in the office have percentages ranging from 35 to 50 percent, and most of the men 33 to 38 percent. Lance Armstrong, when racing, has 4 percent body fat.

For our purposes, I am going to assume that most people, when they finally achieve an ideal weight, will probably Still have a body-fat content around 10 percentage points above the top normal range. Therefore, for our calculations, if they've been significantly overweight for some time, women who have achieved their ideal weight will have a body-fat percentage of approximately 37 percent and men a body-fat percentage of 33 percent.

So if we assume that you're a woman at your ideal weight with a body-fat percentage of 37 percent, then we would multiply your ideal weight by .37. Subtract that result from your total body weight, and you now have your lean body mass. Multiply that number by 12.5, then add to it the number of calories you burn exercising. This can be determined by multiplying your total body weight by 3 if you're sedentary, by 5 if you're moderately active, and by 7.5 if you're very active.

So if your ideal body weight is 150 pounds, and you have 37 percent body fat, then your lean body mass is 94.5 pounds (150 x .37 = 55.5, 150 - 55.5 = 94.5). We multiply this by 12.5, and we get 1,181.

This is how many calories you'll burn per day, not taking activity into account. If you are moderately active, we multiply five times your total body weight and get 750 calories. We add these two numbers together for a total of 1,931 calories. If we divide this number by 5, we end up with about 386 calories for each of the five meals you eat every day. This is not very different from the 350 you started with.

Let's for arguments sake say that you have taken your exercise very seriously. In fact, you're doing some serious weight training, alternating that with some form of aerobic exercise so that you are working out almost every day. To your delight, you recently had your body fat measured, and it turned out to be only 28 percent. Let's refigure your caloric requirements.

A total body weight of 150 x .28 = 42 pounds of fat. 150 - 42 = 108 pounds of lean body mass. 108 x 12.5 = 1,350 is the number of calories you burn every day, regardless of exercise. Add to that the number of calories for exercise you are now getting: 7.5 x 150 = 1,125. Add these two numbers together, and your total caloric requirement to maintain your ideal weight of 150 pounds would be 2,475. If we now divide this by five, we get 495 calories—the number of calories in each of the five small meals that you eat each day.

I give this illustration only to point out what a major difference exercise and building muscle can have on your daily caloric requirements. I certainly would not expect most people to achieve that much exercise dedication, nor am I suggesting even attempting it. I just want you to have a better understanding of the role that exercise does play, and perhaps why losing weight has been more difficult up to now.

So let's run through this exercise for a male whose ideal weight is 180 pounds. With the assumption that his body-fat percentage is 33 percent, his lean body mass would be 121 pounds (rounding off to the nearest whole number). That would be 180 x .33 = 59.4, 180 - 59.4 = 120.6. If we then multiply 121 by 12.5, we arrive at a basic metabolic burn rate of 1,513. If he gets moderate exercise, we multiply 180 by 5, and we get 900 calories. Adding these two numbers together, we arrive at 2,413 calories. Dividing this total by five, we get 482.6—the calorie requirement for each of five meals per day. Again, this is not far off from the original 450 calories we originally started with.

For argument's sake, let's do the reverse of what we did for the female example. Let's suppose he hasn't exercised much at all during this process, since he just hasn't gotten around to it. He has a body-fat percentage of around 38 percent, even though he's managed to arrive at his ideal weight of 180 pounds. We now multiply 180 x .38 to arrive at a body-fat content of 68 pounds. We subtract the 68 pounds from 180 to arrive at a lean body mass of 112. When we multiply this number by 12.5, we get a basic metabolic rate of 1,400 calories per day. Adding to that number the number of calories for exercise, 180 x 4 (somewhere between active and sedentary), we get 720 calories for a total of 2,120 calories per day. Divide this number by five, and he can now only eat 424 calories per meal. Still, this is not far off from the originally suggested 450 calories.

I think by now you can understand why I picked the numbers I did as the ideal place to start for each of your five meals. Hopefully, I have also convinced you of the importance of keeping track of your weight on a regular basis, as it will be required for some fine-tuning of your caloric requirements. Most importantly, I hope I've illustrated how important exercise really is.

The formula below echoes what we have used in the above calculations. Feel free to plug in your own figures.

_____ x _____ = _____
ideal body weight   percent body fat   pounds of body fat

_____ – _____ = _____
ideal body weight   pounds of body fat   lean body mass

_____ x _____12.5_____ = _____
lean body mass   basic calories burned daily

_____ x _____ = _____
ideal body weight   activity level   calories burned by activity

_____ + _____ = _____
basic calories   activity calories   total daily calorie requirement

_____ ÷ _____5_____ = _____
total calories   calories per meal

Let's review our steps.

Step 1: Stop drinking your calories
Step 2: Eat breakfast
Step 3: Eat a small meal between breakfast and lunch
Step 4: Eat an appetizer a few hours before dinner
Step 5: Find exercise that you enjoy.
Step 6: (Part 1) Refine your meals to goal size through the low density method.
Step 6: (Part 2) Refine your meals to goal size through the high protein method.
Step 7: Apply your new-found knowledge to everyday meals.
Step 8: Fine tune your calories.

Chapter Twenty-Six

June 2007

Today was Cheryl's big day. So far, everything was proceeding as smoothly as could be expected.

Cheryl got ready in her dressing room at the estate. Mrs. Curtis insisted on being there and helping; Cheryl was glad. The hairdresser finished with Cheryl's hair and stood back to admire her handiwork. She finally let Cheryl look in the mirror, and Cheryl loved what she saw.

It was time to get into her dress. Teresa got it off the hanger and undid the many buttons in the back of the old-fashioned, lace- and pearl-studded gown. It had a fitted bodice and scooped neck, low enough to suggest the promise of softness, but not so low to be considered revealing. The long narrow sleeves made her arms appear so slender. Cheryl stepped into the dress and pulled it up while others crowded behind to redo all those tiny little buttons. She honestly had trouble believing that the girl staring back from the mirror was really her. Cheryl had pinched herself a few times, and she still wasn't sure it was real. How many changes had taken place in just over two years? It was hard to keep track. When she had entered Dr. Lang's office for the first time, she would not have ever believed that she'd become who she was today.

Time was passing, and everyone drifted away to get to the ceremony as scheduled. Maria took Angelina's hand and carried her basket of flowers for her. Teresa picked up Cheryl's train. Anita made a last adjustment to Cheryl's veil. The music was playing. It was time to go.

Cheryl stood in the back behind a screen, waiting for her cue. As the Wedding March began, adrenaline coursed through her body. She stepped out and slowly walked down the aisle. Victor was there, waiting for her. He looked so handsome in his tuxedo. He smiled, his eyes crinkling and twinkling. She smiled back under her veil.

Cheryl saw Victor's expression sober suddenly; he was looking beyond her. When he looked back at Cheryl, she could visibly see his spirits lift again. *What was that all about?* she wondered, but just as quickly realized that his father must have finally arrived.

The entire ceremony flew by in what seemed like seconds. When the minister gave the go-ahead, Victor kissed her so long that the audience started chuckling out loud. When the newlyweds turned to leave the altar, Victor stumbled on her train but fortunately caught himself. Cheryl smiled at him, and they walked down the aisle, arm in arm, laughing together. The reception was everything Cheryl could have asked for and more. She only wished that it could go on longer. The four hours flew by in what seemed like minutes. They tried to see and greet everyone, but it was an overwhelming task, and before they knew it, people were leaving.

Cheryl had seen Victor talking to his father somewhat heatedly, but then he seemed to calm down. He told her that he had agreed to meet his dad tomorrow at the airport for breakfast before they flew off for their honeymoon. He said his father had apologized for being so late but wanted to explain over breakfast tomorrow.

Cheryl agreed. They were staying at the motel right by the airport tonight, so they'd have no problem making the early flight.

Shortly before the newlyweds were about to leave the reception, one of the estate managers managed to track Cheryl down with an urgent telephone message. Cheryl was to call the convalescent home immediately. Cheryl suddenly didn't feel so well. She expected the worst.

What she didn't expect was the news that her mother was conscious and asking for her.

Cheryl burst into tears. Victor was by her side instantly.

"What's the matter, baby?" He had obviously misunderstood Cheryl's reaction.

Cheryl was so overwhelmed with emotion that she could hardly speak. "It's Mom. She ... she woke up."

"Cheryl, that's wonderful!" Victor picked her up by the waist and twirled her around and around in circles. Cheryl started to laugh, and then Victor joined in. He finally put Cheryl down so they could share a tearful embrace.

"Let's go see her right now!" Victor said.

"Do you think we could? Just like we are? Wouldn't that be wonderful?"

"Yes, of course, just like we are."

So rather than heading for the airport motel, they had the limousine take them to the convalescent home. Cheryl was still in her wedding dress, and Victor in his tux. They entered the convalescent home amid all kinds of stares, but who cared?

When they entered Charlotte's room, they didn't know what to expect. She looked pretty much as she always did, seemingly asleep. But when Cheryl took her hand, she opened her eyes and stared for several moments. Finally, she spoke, "You're so beautiful … and thin! Am I in heaven?"

Cheryl shook her head. Charlotte looked intently at Cheryl's face.

"Cheryl?"

"Yes, Mom."

Charlotte looked at Victor, standing at the foot of the bed. She looked back at Cheryl, and then again at Victor. Understanding dawned. "Oh my G—you're married? Today is your wedding day?"

"Yes, Mom."

"Well … I …" Charlotte struggled for words, then finally said simply, "What a wonderful vision to wake up to."

"And what a wonderful wedding present!" Cheryl exclaimed.

Cheryl leaned over and kissed her mom on the forehead. Her mother squeezed her hand in return. Cheryl turned to Victor. "Honey, I can't leave tomorrow. I hope you can understand."

"Of course; we'll just have to take a delayed honeymoon. That's okay, baby. I understand."

Charlotte looked at them both. "If you don't go on your honeymoon, I will never forgive myself."

"Oh, Mom. I can't."

"You certainly can. And you will. Cheryl Morris …" She paused. "What's your name now?"

Victor answered, "DePalma."

"Cheryl DePalma, I did not wake up today to begin interfering with your life. You will go on your honeymoon, or I'll go right back into a coma. Do you understand?"

Hearing that stubborn voice made Cheryl smile.

"Oh, Mama. I've missed you so much. I just want to spend some time with you."

"You'll have plenty of time to spend with me when you get back. Apparently, I'm not going anywhere. It seems that God has other plans for me."

"But how will I be able to enjoy my honeymoon if I'm worried about you?"

"You'll call me every morning, and I will tell you how wonderfully I'm doing, and then you can enjoy the rest of the day."

Cheryl didn't have any other arguments, and she could see her mother was getting very tired. She was amazed and pleased that she was being so much like her old self.

"Now, you go back to your hotel and consummate your marriage, like you're supposed to, and let me get some rest so I have the energy to talk to you on the phone in the morning."

"Yes, Mama."

Charlotte looked at Victor. "And you take very good care of her, son. You hear?"

"Yes, ma'am. But don't worry, Mrs. Morris. She's very precious to me too."

Charlotte grinned. "Go! Enjoy! I'll talk to you in the morning."

Cheryl and Victor left the room but stopped at the front desk to determine the best times to call in the morning. Cheryl hated to leave, but at the same time, she knew that it didn't make any sense to not abide by her mother's wishes. She supposed if she called every day as planned, she'd be able to deal with her concerns.

They finally arrived at their hotel room at the airport.

"Well, Mrs. DePalma, how does it feel?" Cheryl sat on the edge of the bed and bounced up and down, as though she were testing it out for purchase. They had never stayed in a hotel together before.

"It feels a little … illicit."

Victor laughed. "It does, doesn't it?"

They checked out the closets, the minibar, and the bathroom. While they were looking around, Victor remarked casually, "You know, baby, I was really surprised when you dived into a piece of wedding cake. I've never seen you eat much cake."

"Of course I had to eat a piece of my own wedding cake. How could I not? But did you notice, sweetheart? I ate hardly any dinner."

"Now that I think of it, you didn't really eat much. So that's how you get away with it."

"Dr. Lang calls it intelligent cheating!"

"What do you mean, intelligent cheating?" Victor asked as he checked the thermostat.

"Well, you're not really cheating, but when you follow all the diet principles, it just seems like you're cheating sometimes. If I have a piece of cake instead of a meal, I'm still sticking with five small meals a day. Or if I have a great big piece of roast beef for dinner, but no carbs, then I can get away with it, because I'm doing the Atkins thing. Either way, I'm sticking to the plan."

"Hey, way too complicated for me!" Victor said as he took off his trousers and put them on a hanger. He suggested that Cheryl use the bathroom first, as she was almost undressed already.

She finished in the bathroom and slid into bed as Victor went in to take a shower. She tried to stay awake but couldn't fight the exhaustion. She felt her eyelids drooping. Then she felt Victor slide into bed beside her. He wrapped his arms around her from behind and kissed her on the back of the head.

"Good night, Mrs. DePalma."

"G'night," she murmured.

The following morning, as promised, Cheryl called to talk to her mom. She sounded good. Cheryl was reassured.

At breakfast, Victor's dad explained to Victor and Cheryl what had held him up.

"I'm really so sorry, Victor. I did so want to be there for you, but when I went to the emergency room with chest pain, they kept me there for immediate angioplasty. I didn't want to call for fear of ruining your wedding plans. I hope you understand," Mr. DePalma explained.

"I'm sorry, Dad, for getting so upset with you. I just wish I'd known. Why didn't you tell me any of this before?"

"I don't know. My health just seemed to get out of hand. I've been depressed lately and putting on all this weight. Then my doctor told me I had diabetes, and I had to lose weight. That advice just seemed to make it worse."

Cheryl stared at the plate in front of Victor's father. It held the remains of two eggs, bacon, pancakes, butter, and syrup that had covered the surface from edge to edge. Victor was at a loss for words. He looked at his watch.

"You know, Cheryl, we should be getting on. The plane is getting ready to board."

"Mr. DePalma, I have the name of a doctor who could help you. Wait a minute ... I'll see if I have one of her cards in my purse." Cheryl dug around in her purse for her last appointment card.

"Come on, Cheryl. We really should get going," Victor urged.

"Here," she said, as she handed the card to his father.

"What would you know about any of this? You're so slim and beautiful."

Cheryl, looking up at Victor, smiled and winked. "More than you know," Cheryl said. "More than you know."

As Victor pulled Cheryl away, she called back to Mr. DePalma, "You go see that doctor while you're here in Philadelphia. You won't be sorry."

WEIGHTS AND MEASURES

1 tablespoon (tbsp) =	3 teaspoons (tsp)
1/16 cup =	1 tablespoon (tbsp)
1/8 cup =	2 tablespoons (tbsp)
1/6 cup =	2 tablespoons (tbsp) + 2 teaspoons (tsp)
1/4 cup =	4 tablespoons (tbsp)
1/3 cup =	5 tablespoons (tbsp) + 1 teaspoon (tsp)
3/8 cup =	6 tablespoons (tbsp)
1/2 cup =	8 tablespoons (tbsp)
2/3 cup =	10 tablespoons (tbsp) + 2 teaspoons (tsp)
3/4 cup =	12 tablespoons (tbsp)
1 cup =	48 teaspoons (tsp)
1 cup =	16 tablespoons (tbsp)
8 fluid ounces (fl oz) =	1 cup
1 pint (pt) =	2 cups
1 quart (qt) =	2 pints (pt)
4 cups =	1 quart (qt)
1 gallon (gal) =	4 quarts (qt)
16 ounces (oz) =	1 pound (lb)
1 milliliter (ml) =	1 cubic centimeter (cc)
1 inch (in) =	2.54 centimeters (cm)

U.S. TO METRIC

Capacity	
1/5 teaspoon (tsp)	1 milliliter (ml)
1 teaspoon (tsp)	5 milliliter (ml)
1 tablespoon (tbsp)	15 milliliters (ml)
1 fluid ounce (oz)	30 milliliters (ml)
1/5 cup	47 milliliters (ml)
1 cup	237 milliliters (ml)
2 cups (1 pint (pt))	473 milliliters (ml)
4 cups (1 quart (qt))	.95 liter (l)
4 quarts 1 gallon (gal))	3.8 liters (l)
Weight	
1 ounce (oz)	28 grams (g)
1 pound (lb)	454 grams (g)

METRIC TO U.S.

Capacity	
1 milliliter (ml)	1/5 teaspoon (tsp)
5 milliliter (ml)	1 teaspoon (tsp)
15 milliliter (ml)	1 tablespoon (tbsp)
100 milliliter (ml)	3.4 fluid ounces (fl oz)
240 milliliter (ml)	1 cup
1 liter (l)	34 fluid ounces (fl oz)
	= 4.2 cups

	=2.1 pints (pt)
	=1.06 quarts (qt)
	=0.26 gallon (gal)
Weight	
1 gram (g)	.035 ounce (oz)
100 grams (g)	3.5 ounces (oz)
500 grams (g)	1.10 pounds (lb)
1 kilogram (kg)	2.205 pounds (lb) = 35 ounces (oz)

NUTRIENT WEIGHTS

3,600 calories = one pound

Carbohydrate =	4 calories/gram (g)
Fat =	9 calories/gram (g)
Protein =	4 calories/gram (g)

RECOMMENDED DIETARY ALLOWANCES (RDAS)

RDAs can also be referred to as DRIs (dietary reference intakes)

AI (adequate intake) is listed where no RDA has been established

*Smokers should add 35 mg to these values
μg is the symbol for micrograms
**5 μg = 200 IU (International Units)

	Women (adult)	Men (adult)
Protein	50 g	63 g
Vitamin A (retinal)	700 μg	900 μg
Thiamine (Vitamin B1)	1.1 mg	1.2 mg
Riboflavin (Vitamin B1)	1.1 mg	1.3 mg
Niacin (Vitamin B3)	14 mg	16 mg
Pantothenic acid (VitaminB5)	5 mg (AI)	5 mg (AI)
Vitamin B6	1.3 mg	1.3 mg
Vitamin B12	2.4 μg	2.4 μg
Vitamin C	75 mg*	75 mg*
Vitamin D	5 μg (AI)**	5 μg (AI)**
Vitamin E	15 mg	15 mg
Folacin	400 μg	400 μg
Biotin	30 μg (AI)	30 μg (AI)
Calcium	1,000 mg(AI)	1,000 mg (AI)
Phosphorus	700 mg	700 mg
Selenium	55 μg	70 μg
Iron	18 mg	10 mg
Zinc	8 mg	15 mg
Magnesium	310 mg	400 mg
Iodine	150 μg	150 μg
Fluoride	3 μg	4 μg

CALORIES BURNED BY LEAN BODY MASS

Perhaps you are wondering where I got the figure of 12.5 calories per pound of lean body mass burned daily. You won't find that number anywhere in any literature. Many studies and many articles discuss exactly this subject, but none have found a universally accepted answer. This measurement is very difficult. Lean body mass just eliminates the fat, and then you have to consider everything else. The heart and the kidneys burn a lot more calories per pound than muscle does. The size of your kidneys and heart doesn't change all that much, but as a percentage of your body mass, they do as you lose weight.

Looking at many, many charts and calculations, I arrived at this figure on my own. It may not be absolutely accurate, but for the needs of anyone using this book to lose weight and eat better, it seems to be about right. Some experts might quarrel with this number, but for the most part, it seems to fit the majority of calculations. I am certainly open to additional information that might help us better understand this concept.

Clearly, it is to our advantage to replace fat with muscle, as we definitely burn more calories per day when lean body mass increases and fat body mass decreases, regardless of exercise. How many calories is still the question, but I would venture to say that my number is not far off.

WHAT ARE OMEGA-3 FATTY ACIDS?

Omega-3 fatty acids are polyunsaturated fats that the body is not capable of man-ufacturing. We must obtain them from the foods we eat. These fatty acids appear to encourage the formation of good cholesterol. They also have anti-inflamma-tory effects, as well as anticlotting effects.

These essential fatty acids are found in cold-water fish, including tuna, mack-erel, and salmon; dark green, leafy vegetables; flaxseed oils; canola; and olive oils. Fish oil capsules containing omega-3 fatty acids are available as supplements. Many who are interested in improving their HDL cholesterol can benefit from these supplements.

WHAT ARE TRANS FATTY ACIDS?

Several decades ago, when it was determined that saturated fats were not good for you and polyunsaturated fats were, the food industry came up with a method to help solidify polyunsaturated fats in order to prolong their shelf life by hydroge-nating them. These hydrogenated polyunsaturated fats were termed "trans fatty acids." Unfortunately, over the following years, it became apparent that these trans fatty acids increased both total cholesterol as well as the LDL ("bad" cholesterol). In fact, they were no better than the original saturated fats.

Recently, food manufacturers have been required to label the amount of trans fatty acids found in any given packaged food. This ruling went into full effect in 2006. Most food labels will now alert you to the amount of cholesterol, saturated fats, and trans fats. If you are watching your cholesterol, you particularly want to avoid these fats.

ABOUT GLYCEMIC INDEX AND GLYCEMIC LOAD

Although learning about the glycemic index and the glycemic load of certain foods is not absolutely crucial to healthy eating, it's still important. But like any job well done, the more you know and understand, the more likely you will have greater success.

On the following pages, you will find a clear explanation of "glycemic index" and "glycemic load." Following that is a list of very low-glycemic foods. A complete glycemic index can be found on my Web site, NovelMedicine.info. Use these lists regularly to help make better choices.

The glycemic index (GI) is a number that refers to how rapidly a particular food can raise your blood sugar. To better understand the concept, let me explain how it is calculated. Usually, ten people are given exactly fifty grams of a particular biologically active carbohydrate. Then each of their blood sugars is measured over a short period of time to determine how quickly their blood sugar rises. An average of all the results is then calculated, and a single number is assigned. The quicker the rise in the blood sugar, the higher the number.

You are now probably asking yourself what I mean by "biologically active." Remember when we discussed low-density foods? We established that fiber and water content don't represent a significant calorie count, because fiber is mostly not absorbed by the body, and water has zero calories. Well, when we refer to a biologically active carbohydrate, we are talking about the portion of the carbohydrate that has calories. If we are going to place foods in a meaningful statistical list, it is crucial that we compare the same amount of active ingredient from person to person so that we are not comparing numbers arising from different quantities ingested.

So, for example, if we were to measure 50 grams of carbohydrate in watermelon, that does not mean that the person has to eat 50 grams of watermelon. It means that they have to each eat 750–960 grams of watermelon (approximately three to four 8-ounce slices without the rind) to be eating 50 grams of carbohydrate, since every ounce of watermelon contains about 1.5 to 2 carbs. Put another way, those people would have to eat the equivalent of approximately 4 1/2 to 6 cups of cubed watermelon. (There is no set amount, as some watermelon will have more or less measurable carbohydrate, depending on the amount of water and sweetness. I point this out because when you look up these values in different books, you will find different numbers. The small variation in these numbers should not make a big difference.)

Now, if you tried to measure the glycemic index of lettuce, each person would have to eat twenty cups of shredded lettuce in order to achieve fifty grams of biologically active carbohydrate. To measure celery, they would have to ingest eight cups of cubed celery. It would be unrealistic to try to measure the glycemic index of these foods.

What is obvious even without measurement, though, is that these foods would have very low glycemic indices. They are considered in some circles to be "free foods" with regard to raising the blood sugar. Many other foods have very low or immeasurable glycemic indices. You will find a list of these foods in the following pages.

Glycemic load (GL) refers to the quantity of carbs that will enter the bloodstream from a given serving of a particular food.

Now, we're measuring how much an average serving might raise the blood sugar as opposed to the 50 grams required when measuring the GI . The glycemic load is calculated by multiplying the glycemic index of a particular food by the actual amount of carbohydrate in a serving, then dividing by 100.

To better understand this concept, let's look at the glycemic load of some different foods. Let's begin with our above example, watermelon. Watermelon has a glycemic index of 72. But remember, that was determined by eating 750–960 grams of watermelon. Suppose you eat only four ounces (just under a cup of cubed melon). Then the glycemic load would only be 4 to 6—quite a different number than the glycemic index. Glycemic loads below 10 are considered low, and loads above 20 are considered high.

Baked potatoes contain 6 to 7 carbs per ounce, depending on which reference you read. If we consider a five-ounce baked potato an average serving, then it will have thirty to thirty-five carbs per serving. Its glycemic index is about eighty-five (if served without butter). So if we do the math 85 x 30 divided by 100 we get a glycemic load of approximately twenty-five to thirty. If we add butter to the baked potato, it could reduce the GI to as low as sixty, because fat slows the absorption process (even though it adds a lot of calories). We then find that we have a GL of eighteen to twenty-one. Still not a low number.

On the following pages, you'll find a list of very low-glycemic index foods. On my Web site, NovelMedicine.info, you will find a complete glycemic index. These lists should help you in choosing the right foods.

It's important to understand that low-glycemic index carbohydrates and low-density foods are basically the same types of food. Low-density foods should become a major part of your diet. Some foods, even though they have a high glycemic index, can still be enjoyed on a regular basis, because they have a low glycemic load. By utilizing the lists properly, you can add the right foods to your diet repertoire. Remember, different references will cite different numbers, but low-GI foods will always be low-GI foods. High-GI foods will always be high-GI foods. A slight variation in numbers is not important.

Low-GL foods will only remain low if the portions are controlled. For example, a small amount of watermelon is fine, but a very large portion is not.

The lower the glycemic load, the lower the calorie count. Four ounces of watermelon only has about 24 to 30 calories. Two cups (around ten to eleven ounces) of cubed watermelon has closer to 100 calories.

VERY LOW GLYCEMIC INDEX CARBOHYDRATES

(Suitable to use with low-carb meals)
THAT ARE ALSO VERY LOW-DENSITY FOODS
(Large in volume, low in calories)

Each of the vegetables listed below has less than 5 grams of carbohydrates for each 100 grams (3 1/2 oz) of the food listed. Remember, this is a weight value, not a volume value. The volumes could vary from 1/2 cup (4 "liquid" ounces)* to 2 cups (16 "liquid" ounces)* or even more, depending on the particular vegetable. However, even if you choose a larger volume of any of the foods listed below, the calorie count and the glycemic load will remain quite low.

Alfalfa seeds, sprouted	Artichokes	Avocado**
Arugula	Asparagus, cooked	Bamboo shoots, cooked
Beans, green, cooked	Beans, snap, cooked	Bean sprouts
Bok choy	Beet greens, cooked	Broccoli
Cabbage, cooked	Cauliflower, cooked	Celery
Chard, Swiss, cooked	Chicory, greens	Collards, cooked
Cucumber	Dandelion greens, cooked	Eggplant, cooked
Endive	Fennel, bulb	Hearts of palm, canned
Jicama	Kale, cooked	Lettuce, butterhead
Lettuce, cos or romaine	Lettuce, iceberg	Mung bean, sprouts
Mustard greens, cooked	Mushrooms (not shiitake)	Parsley

---

* I have put the word liquid in quotations to indicate that, although none of these vegetables are liquid, when measuring volumes, we use a measuring cup, and this is the space the vegetable takes up in the cup.

** Not low-density, but has a low glycemic index.

Peppers, serrano	Peppers, jalapeño	Peppers, sweet green
Peppers, sweet red	Pumpkin, cooked	Purslane
Radicchio	Radishes	Rhubarb
Sauerkraut	Scallions (green onions)	Sorrel, raw
Spinach, cooked	Squash, summer, cooked	Squash, zucchini, cooked
Tomatillos	Tomatoes	Turnips, cooked
Turnip greens, cooked	Watercress	

Please visit my Web site, NovelMedicine.info, for a complete glycemic index.

RECIPE SECTION

I debated with myself on many occasions whether to put a recipe section in this book. Since so many excellent cookbooks already offer wonderful low-calorie recipes designed by qualified chefs, I felt any recipes I created would be poor substitutes. But for the sake of helping you design an approach to creating quick, satisfying meals, I decided to offer a few quick sauce recipes, some ingredient suggestions, and a list of cookbooks offering delicious low-cal recipes.

Breakfast Meal Suggestions
- **Cereal**, preferably a high-fiber cereal, with a piece of fruit (either cut up on top or eaten on the way to work).
- **Packaged fruit yogurt,** chosen according to calorie count. Choose a low-fat, lower-calorie yogurt if you also plan to eat cereal and/or fruit. If you choose a higher calorie count, yogurt should be your sole choice for breakfast.
- **Large portion of fresh fruit salad with plain yogurt,** sweetened with Splenda or Nutrasweet.
- **Hot cereal with fruit topping:** oatmeal, Cream of Wheat, or Cream of Rice, topped with fruit (or you may eat the fruit separately, if you prefer).
- **Two eggs with a slice of whole-wheat (low-carb) toast (40 calories per slice) and soy substitute meat:** (Smart Deli puts out various types that are very low in calories).
- **Egg and bacon sandwich,** using low-carb bread at 40 calories per slice, 1 egg scrambled or fried (100 calories), 2 slices of bacon or sausage (150 calories), or 4 slices turkey bacon (140 calories). Sticking to low-carb bread allows you to indulge in regular bacon or sausage. A healthier choice would be to use the soy substitute meat and have a piece of fruit as well.
- **High-fiber toast or bagel with topping:** The high-fiber bagels are very large and contain 280 calories. However, you can cut them into four bagel-shaped pieces, because they are so thick. Eat only half a bagel at a time, saving the other half for a sandwich, or have two separate pieces to top.
  Topping suggestions
  Preserves or apple butter
  Smoked fish
  Salmon

White fish
Kippers
Sardines
Cream cheese
Other cheeses (plus tomatoes, onions, and so on)

- **Omelets or frittatas:** Omelets are folded; frittatas are served flat. Omelets usually have their ingredients in the center; frittatas have the ingredients all mixed in. If you're not good at flipping the eggs over, I suggest cooking a frittata in a cast-iron pan that can be placed in an oven so that you can evenly cook the top and bottom. (You will need to consider the additional calories for any oil or butter in the pan. You may want to use a nonstick pan and cooking spray.) Another method would be to make a container out of aluminum foil, spray it with cooking spray, and bake the frittata mixture in a toaster oven. You will still need to eat it out of the foil, as it will likely stick (not pretty, but functional). Since the two eggs only have approximately 150 calories, you can have fun being creative with the additional 200 or 300 (for a male) calories. You can add a tablespoon of nonfat sour cream to make the eggs lighter and fluffier.
  Ingredients to consider (which you may want to sauté first):
  Chopped mushrooms
  Onions
  Peppers—green, yellow, red, and so on
  Tomatoes
  Spinach or other greens
  Beans or lentils
  Cheese
  Ham or other meats (be careful of volume)
  To make a lunch or dinner frittata, consider adding hot sauce, barbecue sauce, or other spicy ingredients.

Lunch Meal Suggestions

- **Sandwiches** are certainly the mainstay of most lunches. If you choose the low-carb, high-fiber bread as mentioned above (at only 40 calories per slice), then the interior of the sandwich has tremendous leeway. You could even eat two sandwiches, if you keep the calorie count low in the middle. Be careful of wraps. Often, the tortillas are quite large and can contain as many as 190 calories. Low-carb tortillas do exist, and they only have 100 calories.

Smart Beat imitation mayonnaise is only 10 calories per tablespoon. Using lettuce and tomato only adds another 10 or 20 calories, so each sandwich could have another 90 calories—easily accomplished with tuna fish (60 calories/serving). You even have room to add some onion for additional flavor. Use your imagination to create delicious sandwiches to your liking that you can eat at various times of the day.

Additional Ingredients to Consider

Fresh spinach or other greens (arugula, mustard greens, and so on)
Basil
Cucumber
Olives (sliced—one or two can go a long way to add flavor without a lot of calories)
Crumbled blue cheese (again, a very little can go a long way)
Peppers—sour, sweet, hot, or roasted
Carrots, shredded
Cabbage, shredded
Pickles, sweet or sour
Sauces (see sauce recipes.)
Sardines
Salmon, smoked or regular
Kippers
Mackerel
Eggs

Do you like Italian hoagies? Did you ever stop to consider what makes a hoagie appealing? You can make a sandwich with shredded lettuce and onions, very thinly sliced tomatoes, and whatever meat you prefer, and then season it with a tad of oil and vinegar, oregano, garlic powder, salt, and pepper. Add hot peppers if you like. Much of the flavor that you enjoy on a hoagie can be enjoyed on a sandwich made with many fewer calories. Do you have a toaster oven? Have you ever made a melt? Open sandwiches with melted cheese on the top can be delicious and quite filling. You can make a tuna melt, but use only one slice of bread (40 calories). Still, it can be a very hearty one slice. Use half a can of tuna (75 calories) and put tomatoes, cucumber, onions, and hot peppers on it if you like. Add two slices of cheese on top (140 calories). Place in the toaster oven on high. You still have room for an accompanying simple green salad with dressing. If you don't like tuna, try ham or any other ingredients (consider many mentioned above) that taste good with melted cheese.

- **Salads** too play a major role in healthy lunches as well as dinners. Many of the above ingredients can be used to enhance a salad and make it more interesting. Make certain, however, to count all the calories that go into your salad. I've seen salads with as many as 900 calories. Remember to use high-density foods more as flavorings than as major ingredients.

Additional Salad Ingredients

Parmesan or feta cheese
Beans—all kinds
Bean sprouts
Asparagus
Artichoke hearts
Endive
Corn
Hearts of palm

Dinner Meal Suggestions

Dinner should be a time to sit down and relax and have a full meal. Creating a complete meal with fewer than 350 or 450 calories is not as difficult as it may first seem.

Beginning the meal with a cup of clear soup, such as a mushroom consommé or vegetable soup (30–75 calories), can take the edge off your appetite. Follow that with a salad made primarily of leafy vegetables and low-calorie dressing, or just vinegar or lemon juice (50 calories). By the time you get to the main course, you shouldn't be very hungry.

The small portion of protein (size of the palm of your hand) should be less than 200 calories, which still leaves room for a large portion of low-density vegetables or two smaller portions of two different vegetables (about 25 calories each). If you leave off the soup or salad, you can manage a small portion of starch (rice, potatoes, pasta) in place of one of the vegetables.

The following is a list of sauce recipes to put on any form of protein to make it more interesting. All are generally less than thirty calories and can be made in about five minutes. They are designed to go on top of already-cooked protein—or vegetables that have been baked, broiled, or sautéed—in order to make a boring meal into one that is far more interesting and varied. For convenience, each recipe is for one serving. You can double everything for two servings.

SAUCES

CURRY SAUCE

1 tbsp low-calorie mayonnaise (Smart Beat has only 10 calories per tbsp)
1/8 tsp curry powder
1/8 tsp cumin (if you don't have cumin, use another 1/8 tsp of curry powder.)
1/8 tsp garlic powder
1/8 tsp onion powder
1/16 tsp or less of cayenne pepper (if you don't like things spicy, still use a pinch of cayenne anyway)
Juice from a wedge of lemon (4 or 5 drops of concentrated lemon juice)

Mix the above ingredients together, then serve hot or cold. To heat, put it in the microwave for 20 seconds. Do not cook the sauce with the food; simply warm it in the microwave and put it on the already cooked food you plan to eat with it. Tasty with chicken, pork, or vegetables.

HORSERADISH SAUCE

1 tbsp low-calorie mayonnaise
1 tbsp horseradish (you can find jars of horseradish in the refrigerated dairy section of the supermarket)
Few drops of Worcestershire sauce
Few drops of lemon juice

Mix the above ingredients and serve hot or cold. This sauce is great with seafood.

RUSSIAN DRESSING/SAUCE

1 heaping tbsp of low-calorie mayonnaise
3/4 tsp ketchup
1 tsp relish
1/8 tsp garlic powder
1/8 tsp dill
Few drops lemon juice
Fresh ground pepper to taste

Mix and serve, hot or cold.

ORANGE MUSTARD SAUCE

1 rounded tsp dark mustard

1 rounded tsp orange marmalade (you can substitute any flavored preserve you prefer)

Mix well and put on top of fish, chicken, or pork. Unlike other sauce recipes made with mayonnaise, this sauce can be put on the food before baking or broiling.

HONEY MUSTARD SAUCE
1 rounded tsp low-calorie mayonnaise
1 rounded tsp dark mustard
1/4 pack of Splenda
Juice from a lemon wedge

Mix the ingredients well, then microwave for 20 seconds before serving. Great on chicken, fish, or pork, as well as many vegetables.

BLUE CHEESE SAUCE/DRESSING
1 tbsp nonfat sour cream
1 tsp (exact, not heaping) blue cheese (soften in the microwave for 10 or 15 seconds for easier mixing)
1/8 tsp onion powder
1/2 tsp dried chives
Few drops of lemon juice
Salt and pepper to taste

Mix well and serve. To use as a dressing, you may want to double the recipe and add 1–2 tablespoons of water. If you are a blue-cheese lover, this sauce goes well on almost anything.

Cheese Sauce
1 heaping tbsp low-calorie mayonnaise
3/4 tbsp of grated Parmesan cheese
1/8 tsp fresh ground pepper
1/8 tsp garlic powder

Mix well, and heat in the microwave for 20 seconds. Put on vegetables or chicken.

Peanut Sauce
1 tbsp nonfat sour cream

1 rounded tsp reduced-fat peanut butter
1/8 tsp sesame oil
Scant 1/8 tsp cayenne pepper
1/8 tsp garlic powder
1/8 tsp rice or cider vinegar
Dash of salt
Pinch of Splenda

Mix together and heat in microwave. Very nice on chicken, pork, and some vegetables.

Sweet Chile Sauce
1 tbsp rice or cider vinegar
1 tbsp water
1/4 tsp garlic powder
Scant 1/8 tsp cayenne
3/16 tsp of Splenda (if using 1/8 tsp measure, use 1 1/2 of these)
1 tsp lemon juice
1/8 tsp xanthan gum (You can find xanthan gum in the health-food store)

Mix with a handheld blender for about one minute.
This sauce is something like the duck sauce that you get at Chinese restaurants, only a bit spicier. You can, of course, leave out the cayenne if you prefer.

- **Stir-fry** is another type of dinner to consider. Cutting a portion of protein into small, bite-size pieces allows it to go much further. Sautéing it with a multitude of vegetables with various spices and oils can change the flavor significantly.
  Sesame oil (use just 1–2 tsp in a nonstick pan) gives a distinctive Asian flavor. Asian vegetables can also add great variety—try water chestnuts, bamboo shoots, bean sprouts, and miniature corn. A bit of soy, some Splenda (yes, there is a fair amount of sugar in Chinese stir-fry), and some garlic powder will give a more authentic Chinese flavor. If you like spicy, add some chili peppers. If you keep the protein amount small, then you can use store-bought oyster sauce (which has little to do with oysters) and is a familiar Chinese food flavoring.
  Stir-fry does not have to have the above flavoring. Lemon, garlic, and oregano will give it a more Italian flavor. Use your imagination to come

up with your own style. Barbecue sauce could be used as well. Anything goes when you're the chef.

- **Fajitas** are another option, if you keep the protein portion small. Low-carb tortillas are available at only 100 calories, with 7 grams of fiber. Sauté onions and peppers (or other vegetables) along with your protein of choice (leftovers are great, whether it's chicken, turkey, pork, or beef), then add your store-bought sauce mix. Place several tablespoons of the mixture into warmed tortillas, and fold. Serve with nonfat sour cream and taco sauce. Avoid guacamole—too many additional calories.

- **Pizzas** can be made using these same tortillas for the crust. Place the tortilla in the toaster oven on medium toast to crisp it up just a little. Smear a little tomato sauce all over the tortilla. Add mushrooms, spinach, onions, or whatever you prefer. Smart Deli makes a substitute pepperoni, or you can use turkey pepperoni, which will keep the calorie count low. Season with garlic powder, pepper, oregano, and basil. Use low-fat mozzarella, half regular and half nonfat, or Smart Balance imitation mozzarella. (This brand is good if you're watching your cholesterol.) Sprinkle your pizza with some Parmesan cheese, and toast it in the toaster oven on high. Serve with salad.

Hopefully, by now you have some ideas to get you started. Don't be afraid to make mistakes; that's how you learn. Become more aware of what you're eating and what flavors appeal to you so that you can learn what to use when you're improvising. Keep trying new foods, new meals, and different ways of cooking. Each time you find a great meal, don't forget to repeat it often so it becomes a real habit.

Below is a list of some low-calorie cookbooks. You also may want to subscribe to a cooking magazine, such as *Cooking Light* or *Eating Well.* That way, each month (or every other month), you will have the opportunity to look at some new ideas, complete with photographs, to help spice up your imagination.

365 Easy Low-Calorie Recipes by Sylvia Schur and Vivian Schulte

Southern Living: Our Best Low-Fat, Low-Calorie Recipes, Jean Wickstrom Wiles (Compiler) and Lisa Hooper Talley (Editor)

Good Morning America Cut the Calories Cookbook: 120 Low-Fat, Low-Calorie Recipes from Our Viewers, Jean Anderson and Sara Moulton

Cooking Light Annual Recipes 2005, Heather Averett (Editor)

The Best of Cooking Light, Holley Contri Johnson (Compiler)

The Complete Cooking Light Cookbook, Cathy A. Wesler (Compiler)

Cooking Light Annual Recipes 2004, Mary Kay Culpepper (Editor)
Superfast Suppers: Speedy Solutions for Dinner Dilemmas, Anne C. Cain *(Cooking Light)*
5 Ingredient 15-Minute Cookbook: Cooking Light, Anne Chappell Cain
Five-Star Recipes: The Best of Ten Years (Cooking Light)
Lose Weight Cookbook, Susan McIntosh *(Cooking Light)*
Quick and Easy Cookbook, Susan McIntosh *(Cooking Light)*
Low-Fat Low Calorie: Quick and Easy Cookbook, by Leisure Arts *(Cooking Light)*
Cooking Light the Lazy Gourmet (Cooking Light)
Six Ingredients or Less: Cooking Light and Healthy, Carlean Johnson
Stir-Fry Cookbook, Susan McIntosh *(Cooking Light)*

Of course, many, many other very good cookbooks provide low-calorie recipes. These are possibly some of the better ones. If you have access to a computer, you can find listings for hundreds, if not thousands. Use Amazon.com or Borders.com or any other online book dealer—or just your local bookstore—to find something that fits your fancy.

Better yet, if you have access to a computer, there is no need to purchase any cookbooks. Instead, get your recipes online through the same type of search.

For example, let's say you've just purchased a yellow squash for the first time and would like to find a recipe that has ingredients that appeal to you. Just go to www.google.com and type in "yellow squash." The first listing you'll see is cooks. com. Click on that, and you will be confronted with over 2,000 recipes for yellow squash. Scroll through those recipes until you find one that has most of the ingredients that you like, print it out, and try it. Don't like it? Try another. The Internet is a wonderful source of recipes for just about anything.

I hope I've given you some incentive to venture out and try new foods—and new ways to cook foods you're already familiar with. Being creative can be fun, but also extremely useful in helping you to succeed in your healthy eating endeavor. Be bold, be daring, be adventuresome, and be healthy!

Please find additional meals and recipes on my Web site, NovelMedicine.info.

GLOSSARY

Calorie—The amount of energy required to raise the temperature of 1 gram of water 1 degree centigrade. The measure of energy used in the body.

Carbohydrate—Compounds that are produced by photosynthetic plants and contain only carbon, hydrogen, and oxygen. Any food that's not a protein or a fat.[1]

Complex carbohydrates are chains of simple sugars. They include starches and fiber.

Simple carbohydrates are sugars, including glucose, fructose, galactose, and sucrose.

Diabetes—A disease state causing increased sugar (glucose) levels in the bloodstream.[2]

Glucose—A simple sugar to which most foods are broken down in order for the body for use as energy.

Glycemic index—A number that refers to how rapidly a particular food can raise your blood sugar.[3]

Glycemic load—A number that refers to the quantity of sugar that will enter the bloodstream with a given serving of a particular food.[4]

Gram—A metric unit of measure equal to 1/1,000 of a kilogram. The unit of measure used to quantify fats, proteins, and carbohydrates in food.

HDL cholesterol—Otherwise known as the "good" cholesterol. Stands for high-density lipoprotein.[2]

---

1   See page 140 in the text for a more thorough explanation.
2   See a more complete explanation on my Web site, NovelMedicine.info.
3   See page 239 in the appendix for a more thorough explanation.
4   See page 240 in the appendix for a more thorough explanation.

Hydrogenated fats—Vegetable oils that are chemically treated (hydrogenated) to render them solid at room temperature. Also known as trans fats.[5]

Insulin—A hormone secreted by the pancreas functioning in the regulation of the metabolism/absorption and storage of glucose and fat.

Ketone—A by-product of fat metabolism that can be used as energy by the body. Increased levels of ketones appear to decrease appetite.

LDL cholesterol—Also known as the "bad cholesterol." Stands for low-density lipoprotein.[2]

Low-carb diet—A diet that is composed mostly of protein and fat and contains very few carbohydrates.

Low-density foods—Generally, foods that have a very high fiber and water content so that the amount of calories (energy) per given volume is very small.[6]

Metabolism—The physical and chemical processes occurring within a living cell or organism that is necessary for the maintenance of life.

Anabolism—The phase of metabolism in which simple substances are synthesized into the complex materials of living tissue.

Catabolism—The metabolic breakdown of complex molecules into simpler ones.

Monosaturated fats—Fats that are generally liquid at room temperature. Many are found on the list of foods that help improve HDL cholesterol.

Omega-3 fatty acid—An essential, beneficial fatty acids that cannot be manufactured by the body.[5]

Polyunsaturated fats—Fats that are generally liquid at room temperature. They include safflower, corn, sunflower, and soybean oils. They do tend to lower LDL cholesterol, but, unlike monosaturated fats, do not increase HDL.

---

5   See page 238 in the appendix for a more complete information.

6   See page 97 in the text for additional information.

Protein—The fundamental components of all living cells. They are composed of chains of amino acids and contain carbon, hydrogen, nitrogen, and usually sulfur.[7]

RDA—Recommended daily allowances.

RDI—Recommended daily intakes.

Salmonella—A bacteria that is usually pathogenic, causing food poisoning, typhoid, and typhoid fever. It is most commonly found on chickens.

Sauté—To fry lightly in fat in a shallow, open pan.

Saturated fats—Fats that are generally solid at room temperature. They come mostly from meat. They tend to cause an increase in the "bad" LDL cholesterol.

Starches—Foods composed mainly of chains of simple sugars that are quickly converted into sugar in the stomach, thereby raising blood sugar fairly rapidly.

Sugar alcohol—Sweeteners that are only partially absorbed by the body, so they have fewer calories than standard sugar.[8]

Sweetbreads—The thymus or pancreas glands from calves or young cows.

Trans fatty acids—Liquid vegetable oils that are chemically treated (hydrogenated) so that they are solid at room temperature.[5]

Trichinosis—A disease caused by eating undercooked pork that contains the trichinae larvae. These larvae are easily eliminated by cooking the meat to a temperature greater than 137 degrees Fahrenheit.

---

7   See page 140 in the text for additional information.
8   See page 132 in the text for additional information.

FREQUENTLY ASKED QUESTIONS

Can you really do Atkins two days a week and lose extra weight?

Yes, it will work—with certain caveats. One of the mistakes that many people make upon finishing my book is to focus on one solution to their weight problem—the same thing they've been doing for years. If you don't first change some of your habits to speed up your metabolism, then doing Atkins only two days a week may slow your metabolism even further.

I tried eating five small meals a day and gained weight. Why didn't it work for me?

There might be several reasons. Remember the study that compared two groups of people eating the same amount of calories, but one group in five meals and one group in two meals? When you switched to the five meals, you may have inadvertently started eating more calories than you were eating in two or three meals. Also, some patients have been dieting in one way or another for so long that they have lost so much muscle mass that their metabolism only requires 1,200–1,400 calories per day to maintain their present weight.

I have only been eating 1,200 calories per day for almost a full year, and I can't lose a single pound. Why?

Clearly, your metabolism has been greatly slowed. In my office, I have encountered a number of women with this dilemma. One young lady told me she even went to the gym every day, but upon examination and measurement, she had far more body fat than expected. All her exercise was aerobic exercise. Yes, she was burning calories at the gym, but not building muscle. A scale that measures body fat is not expensive. After measuring your body fat, try to come up with a reasonable exercise program that is aimed at building muscle, then measure your body fat regularly. Begin eating five small meals a day, each one approximately 300 calories. The goal, initially, is not to gain any weight. As you gain lean body mass and your body fat decreases, you should begin to lose weight. You must put your emphasis on changes in body fat in order to accomplish your goal. Once your metabolism begins to improve, but not until that time, you can speed up further weight loss with *intermittent* low-carb or low-calorie restriction.

I'm not the kind of person who can eat five meals a day. Is it really that important?

If you've been trying to lose weight for some time and have been unsuccessful or have succeeded only to gain it back again, then yes, those frequent little meals are very important. These meals

1. Increase your metabolism.
2. Prevent you from getting really hungry.
3. Help prevent unhealthy snacking.
4. Generally keep you in tune with your body.

Yes, change is difficult, but everyone is capable of eating frequent, small meals, regardless of career. You just need to use your intelligence to figure out how to make it happen, rather than rationalizing why you can't.

I always start out with good intentions, but after several weeks or a month, I lose my enthusiasm and end up right back where I started. What can I do to keep it going?

That is exactly why I wrote this book. You need to take it step by step, giving yourself time to develop habits. That way, when your enthusiasm wanes, or you get too stressed to pay attention, you won't end up where you started. Remember Cheryl. She too had her ups and downs, but backsliding was minimal, because she had actually changed a number of habits. If you fall off the habit wagon, before berating yourself, stop and consider what habits still remain. Are you still not drinking your calories? Are you eating breakfast most of the time? Are you eating more meals than when you started? Make sure you give yourself credits for the habits you *have* changed.

Take baby steps. Remember, it took Cheryl over two years to lose all that weight. She didn't even start exercising until several months after she began drinking diet sodas. Make it easy for yourself. Take it slow, and just make sure that each step you take is a correct one.

My girlfriend and I eat almost the same things, and yet she's slim and I'm not—I just don't get it!

Clearly, you have significantly more body fat than your girlfriend. Remember, your basic metabolism (calories burned without additional exercise) is calculated by multiplying your lean body mass by 12.5.* Let's, for argument's sake, say that you weigh 180 pounds, and your girlfriend weighs 140, and your respective body-fat percentages are 40 percent and 20 percent. That means that your lean body mass is 108 pounds (180- (180 x .40)), and your girlfriend's lean body mass is 112 pounds (140- (140 x .20)). So you're burning 1,350 calories without any exercise, and she's burning 1,400 calories. Your basic metabolic requirements are practically the same, even though you weigh 40 pounds more. That's why it is so important to reduce your body-fat percentage through muscle-building exercise.

---

* See further explanation on page 237 of the Appendix.

Is it possible to lose weight without exercising?

Of course you can lose weight without exercise. The effectiveness of dieting without exercise will be greatly dependent on your starting body fat content. I've always been jealous of men who could seemingly lose weight without much effort. In their twenties and thirties, men have significantly more muscle mass than women. But as they age, they too can develop large amounts of body fat. As your body fat content rises, you begin to reach a point of diminishing returns—like the young woman mentioned earlier who was only eating 1,200 calories per day. If you need to eat so few calories in order to eat less than your body burns, you're barely eating enough to maintain your present lean body mass, and you will continue to lose muscle. You may not literally increase your fat stores, but as your muscle mass declines, your body-fat percentage increases.

I eat very healthy organic food, and I'm practically a vegetarian. Why do I still have trouble avoiding weight gain?

All that healthy, organic food obviously comprises more calories than your body burns. Be careful of caloric intake, and follow the basic tenets of this book. Pure organic fruit juice may be healthy with lots of vitamins and minerals, but it can have as many or more calories than soda. Drinking your calories does little to satisfy your appetite, as we have already discussed. Eating to be thin is not the same as eating to be healthy! Nor would I suggest that thin people are necessarily healthier than those who are overweight. Look at Cheryl's mother. Her diseased lungs and failing heart kept her thin. I wouldn't call her healthy. I've known many smokers and alcoholics who were thin and ate incredible amounts of junk food. By the same token, as you have illustrated, you can eat all healthy food and still overeat. One can reduce caloric intake by eating fewer calories, but those calories may not necessarily come from healthy foods. Diet soda is not particularly healthy, but when one is first learning to avoid drinking calories, it is an appropriate choice. A healthier choice would be water.

Remember, climbing a ladder one rung at a time is simpler than jumping to the top. Small, easy modifications allow you to establish better habits and then slowly build on these changes. Once you've learned how acquired taste works and have established a regimen that allows you to maintain a normal weight, you can then go on to make further changes toward a healthier diet, if you so desire.

You can find further FAQs (frequently asked questions) on my Web site, NovelMedicine.info.

978-0-595-44451-9
0-595-44451-2